DASH Delights, a DASH Diet Guide & Cookbook

A Comprehensive Guide on Heart Health and Heart-Healthy Recipes for Lowering Blood Pressure and Weight Management

Plus

BONUS
60-Day Meal Plan to Get You Started

Leopold Knight

Copyright

Disclaimer

The purpose of this book is to provide general information only and not medical advice. It does not replace professional medical advice, diagnosis, or treatment. Always consult your doctor or other qualified health provider if you have any questions about a medical condition. The author and publisher are not responsible for any harm or loss related to recipes in this book.

Bonus

Here is your bonus; 60-day meal plan to get you started on the DASH diet journey, Goodluck!

Day 1
- Breakfast: Spinach & Egg Scramble with Raspberries
- Lunch: Vegan Smoothie Bowl
- Dinner: Slow-Cooker Chicken & White Bean Stew
- Snack: Homemade Trail Mix

Day 2
- Breakfast: Raspberry Yogurt Cereal Bowl
- Lunch: Mason Jar Power Salad with Chickpeas & Tuna
- Dinner: Chickpea & Quinoa Grain Bowl
- Snack: Blueberry Almond Chia Pudding

Day 3
- Breakfast: Chocolate-Banana Protein Smoothie
- Lunch: Sweet Potato, Kale & Chicken Salad with Peanut Dressing
- Dinner: Peppery Barbecue-Glazed Shrimp with Vegetables & Orzo
- Snack: Avocado Hummus

Day 4
- Breakfast: Overnight Quinoa Pudding
- Lunch: Tomato, Cucumber & White-Bean Salad with Basil Vinaigrette
- Dinner: White Turkey Chili
- Snack: Air-Fryer Sweet Potato Chips

Day 5

- Breakfast: Mango-Ginger Smoothie
- Lunch: Rainbow Grain Bowl with Cashew Tahini Sauce
- Dinner: Chicken & Cucumber Lettuce Wraps with Peanut Sauce
- Snack: Apricot-Sunflower Granola Bars

Day 6

- Breakfast: Blueberry-Banana Overnight Oats
- Lunch: Superfood Chopped Salad with Salmon & Creamy Garlic Dressing
- Dinner: Cauliflower Fajita Skillet
- Snack: Zucchini Mini Muffins

Day 7

- Breakfast: Peanut Butter Protein Overnight Oats
- Lunch: Mixed Greens with Lentils & Sliced Apple
- Dinner: Chicken Kebabs with Warm Cabbage-Apple Slaw & Potatoes
- Snack: Rosemary-Garlic Pecans

Day 8

- Breakfast: Breakfast Blueberry-Oatmeal Cakes
- Lunch: Lentil Stew with Salsa Verde
- Dinner: Slow-Cooker Chicken & White Bean Stew
- Snack: Apricot-Ginger Energy Balls

Day 9

- Breakfast: Blueberry Almond Chia Pudding
- Lunch: Chicken & Shredded Brussels Sprout Salad with Bacon Vinaigrette
- Dinner: White Bean Soup with Pasta
- Snack: Avocado-Yogurt Dip

Day 10

- Breakfast: Homemade Plain Greek Yogurt
- Lunch: Quinoa, Avocado & Chickpea Salad over Mixed Greens
- Dinner: Maple-Roasted Chicken Thighs with Sweet Potato Wedges and Brussels Sprouts
- Snack: Air-Fryer Plantains

Day 11

- Breakfast: Banana-Cocoa Soy Smoothie
- Lunch: Smoked Salmon Salad Nicoise
- Dinner: Stuffed Eggplant with Couscous & Almonds
- Snack: Blueberry Almond Chia Pudding

Day 12

- Breakfast: Strawberry & Yogurt Parfait
- Lunch: Chicken with Spinach & Tomato Orzo Salad
- Dinner: Chipotle Chicken Quinoa Burrito Bowl
- Snack: Air-Fryer Sweet Potato Chips

Day 13

- Breakfast: Air-Fryer Crispy Chickpeas
- Lunch: Slow-Cooker Chicken & White Bean Stew
- Dinner: Four-Bean & Pumpkin Chili
- Snack: Apricot-Sunflower Granola Bars

Day 14

- Breakfast: Rice Cake Snackwich
- Lunch: Chicken & Mushroom Ragu
- Dinner: Stuffed Sweet Potato with Hummus Dressing
- Snack: Avocado Hummus

Day 15

- Breakfast: Sprouted-Grain Toast with Peanut Butter & Banana
- Lunch: Tomato, Cucumber & White-Bean Salad with Basil Vinaigrette
- Dinner: Slow-Cooker Chicken Marsala
- Snack: Peanut Butter-Banana Cinnamon Toast

Day 16

- Breakfast: Tasty Guacamole
- Lunch: White Bean & Veggie Salad
- Dinner: Chicken & Sun-Dried Tomato Orzo
- Snack: Rosemary-Garlic Pecans

Day 17

- Breakfast: Kale Chips
- Lunch: Chicken & Cucumber Lettuce Wraps with Peanut Sauce
- Dinner: Sheet-Pan Chili-Lime Salmon with Potatoes & Peppers
- Snack: Banana & Walnut

Day 18

- Breakfast: Mango-Ginger Smoothie
- Lunch: Lentil Stew with Salsa Verde
- Dinner: Provençal Baked Fish with Roasted Potatoes & Mushrooms
- Snack: Air-Fryer Plantains

Day 19

- Breakfast: Peanut Butter Protein Overnight Oats
- Lunch: Mason Jar Power Salad with Chickpeas & Tuna
- Dinner: Chicken & Sun-Dried Tomato Orzo
- Snack: Homemade Trail Mix up

Day 20

- Breakfast: Blueberry Almond Chia Pudding
- Lunch: Slow-Cooked Ranch Chicken and Vegetables
- Dinner: Peppery Barbecue-Glazed Shrimp with Vegetables & Orzo
- Snack: Zucchini Mini Muffins

Day 21

- Breakfast: Banana-Cocoa Soy Smoothie
- Lunch: Quinoa, Avocado & Chickpea Salad over Mixed Greens
- Dinner: Chicken & Mushroom Ragu
- Snack: Avocado-Yogurt Dip

Day 22

- Breakfast: Strawberry-Chocolate Smoothie
- Lunch: Mixed Greens with Lentils & Sliced Apple
- Dinner: Chicken Kebabs with Warm Cabbage-Apple Slaw & Potatoes
- Snack: Rosemary-Garlic Pecans

Day 23

- Breakfast: Breakfast Blueberry-Oatmeal Cakes
- Lunch: Lentil Stew with Salsa Verde
- Dinner: Slow-Cooker Chicken & White Bean Stew
- Snack: Apricot-Sunflower Granola Bars

Day 24

- Breakfast: Blueberry-Banana Overnight Oats
- Lunch: Vegan Superfood Grain Bowl
- Dinner: Cauliflower Fajita Skillet
- Snack: Zucchini Mini Muffins

Day 25

- Breakfast: Spinach & Egg Scramble with Raspberries
- Lunch: Mason Jar Power Salad with Chickpeas & Tuna
- Dinner: Four-Bean & Pumpkin Chili
- Snack: Homemade Trail Mix

Day 26

- Breakfast: Raspberry Overnight Muesli
- Lunch: Chicken with Spinach & Tomato Orzo Salad
- Dinner: Maple-Roasted Chicken Thighs with Sweet Potato Wedges and Brussels Sprouts
- Snack: Banana & Walnut

Day 27

- Breakfast: Mango-Ginger Smoothie
- Lunch: White Bean & Veggie Salad
- Dinner: Chipotle Chicken Quinoa Burrito Bowl
- Snack: Apricot-Ginger Energy Balls

Day 28

- Breakfast: Raspberry Yogurt Cereal Bowl
- Lunch: Spinach & Strawberry Meal-Prep Salad
- Dinner: Spaghetti Squash with Roasted Tomatoes, Beans & Almond Pesto
- Snack: Air-Fryer Sweet Potato Chips

Day 29

- Breakfast: Blueberry Almond Chia Pudding
- Lunch: Mixed Greens with Lentils & Sliced Apple
- Dinner: Chicken & Cucumber Lettuce Wraps with Peanut Sauce
- Snack: Avocado-Yogurt Dip

Day 30

- Breakfast: Overnight Quinoa Pudding
- Lunch: Chickpea & Quinoa Grain Bowl
- Dinner: Slow-Cooker Chicken & White Bean Stew
- Snack: Rosemary-Garlic Pecans

Day 31

- Breakfast: Banana-Cocoa Soy Smoothie
- Lunch: Vegan Smoothie Bowl
- Dinner: Stuffed Sweet Potato with Hummus Dressing
- Snack: Blueberry Almond Chia Pudding

Day 32

- Breakfast: Raspberry Yogurt Cereal Bowl
- Lunch: Slow-Cooked Ranch Chicken and Vegetables
- Dinner: Provençal Baked Fish with Roasted Potatoes & Mushrooms
- Snack: Air-Fryer Sweet Potato Chips

Day 33

- Breakfast: Chocolate-Banana Protein Smoothie
- Lunch: Superfood Chopped Salad with Salmon & Creamy Garlic Dressing
- Dinner: White Turkey Chili
- Snack: Avocado Hummus

Day 34

- Breakfast: Overnight Quinoa Pudding
- Lunch: Tomato, Cucumber & White-Bean Salad with Basil Vinaigrette
- Dinner: Chickpea & Roasted Red Pepper Lettuce Wraps with Tahini Dressing
- Snack: Apricot-Ginger Energy Balls

Day 35

- Breakfast: Mango-Ginger Smoothie
- Lunch: Chicken & Cucumber Lettuce Wraps with Peanut Sauce
- Dinner: Maple-Roasted Chicken Thighs with Sweet Potato Wedges and Brussels Sprouts
- Snack: Homemade Trail Mix

Day 36

- Breakfast: Blueberry-Banana Overnight Oats
- Lunch: Spinach & Strawberry Meal-Prep Salad
- Dinner: Chipotle Chicken Quinoa Burrito Bowl
- Snack: Zucchini Mini Muffins

Day 37

- Breakfast: Peanut Butter Protein Overnight Oats
- Lunch: White Bean & Veggie Salad
- Dinner: Chicken & Sun-Dried Tomato Orzo
- Snack: Apricot-Sunflower Granola Bars

Day 38

- Breakfast: Blueberry Almond Chia Pudding
- Lunch: Lentil Stew with Salsa Verde
- Dinner: Slow-Cooker Chicken & White Bean Stew
- Snack: Avocado-Yogurt Dip

Day 39

- Breakfast: Homemade Plain Greek Yogurt
- Lunch: Quinoa, Avocado & Chickpea Salad over Mixed Greens
- Dinner: Cauliflower Fajita Skillet
- Snack: Banana & Walnut

Day 40

- Breakfast: Raspberry Overnight Muesli
- Lunch: Mason Jar Power Salad with Chickpeas & Tuna
- Dinner: Four-Bean & Pumpkin Chili
- Snack: Rosemary-Garlic Pecans

Day 41

- Breakfast: Breakfast Blueberry-Oatmeal Cakes
- Lunch: Lentil Stew with Salsa Verde
- Dinner: Slow-Cooker Chicken & White Bean Stew
- Snack: Apricot-Sunflower Granola Bars

Day 42

- Breakfast: Blueberry Almond Chia Pudding
- Lunch: Chicken & Shredded Brussels Sprout Salad with Bacon Vinaigrette
- Dinner: White Bean Soup with Pasta
- Snack: Avocado-Yogurt Dip

Day 43

- Breakfast: Tasty Guacamole
- Lunch: Mixed Greens with Lentils & Sliced Apple
- Dinner: Chicken Kebabs with Warm Cabbage-Apple Slaw & Potatoes
- Snack: Rosemary-Garlic Pecans

Day 44

- Breakfast: Kale Chips
- Lunch: Chicken & Cucumber Lettuce Wraps with Peanut Sauce
- Dinner: Sheet-Pan Chili-Lime Salmon with Potatoes & Peppers
- Snack: Banana & Walnut

Day 45

- Breakfast: Mango-Ginger Smoothie
- Lunch: White Bean & Veggie Salad
- Dinner: Chipotle Chicken Quinoa Burrito Bowl
- Snack: Apricot-Ginger Energy Balls

Day 46

- Breakfast: Peanut Butter Protein Overnight Oats
- Lunch: Mason Jar Power Salad with Chickpeas & Tuna
- Dinner: Chicken & Sun-Dried Tomato Orzo
- Snack: Zucchini Mini Muffins

Day 47

- Breakfast: Blueberry Almond Chia Pudding
- Lunch: Slow-Cooked Ranch Chicken and Vegetables
- Dinner: Peppery Barbecue-Glazed Shrimp with Vegetables & Orzo
- Snack: Air-Fryer Sweet Potato Chips

Day 48

- Breakfast: Sprouted-Grain Toast with Peanut Butter & Banana
- Lunch: Tomato, Cucumber & White-Bean Salad with Basil Vinaigrette
- Dinner: Provençal Baked Fish with Roasted Potatoes & Mushrooms
- Snack: Avocado Hummus

Day 49

- Breakfast: Fresh Fruit Salad
- Lunch: Quinoa Power Salad
- Dinner: Lemony Linguine with Spring Vegetables
- Snack: Rosemary-Garlic Pecans

Day 50

- Breakfast: White Bean & Avocado Toast
- Lunch: Beer-Battered Fish Tacos with Tomato & Avocado Salsa
- Dinner: Slow-Cooker Chicken Marsala
- Snack: Air-Fryer Plantains

Day 51

- Breakfast: Lentil Stew with Salsa Verde
- Lunch: Vegan Smoothie Bowl
- Dinner: Stuffed Sweet Potato with Hummus Dressing
- Snack: Blueberry Almond Chia Pudding

Day 52

- Breakfast: Blueberry-Banana Overnight Oats
- Lunch: Superfood Chopped Salad with Salmon & Creamy Garlic Dressing
- Dinner: Cauliflower Fajita Skillet
- Snack: Zucchini Mini Muffins

Day 53

- Breakfast: Mango-Ginger Smoothie
- Lunch: Chicken & Shredded Brussels Sprout Salad with Bacon Vinaigrette
- Dinner: Maple-Roasted Chicken Thighs with Sweet Potato Wedges and Brussels Sprouts
- Snack: Homemade Trail Mix

Day 54

- Breakfast: Peanut Butter Protein Overnight Oats
- Lunch: Tomato, Cucumber & White-Bean Salad with Basil Vinaigrette
- Dinner: Chickpea & Roasted Red Pepper Lettuce Wraps with Tahini Dressing
- Snack: Apricot-Sunflower Granola Bars

Day 55

- Breakfast: Tasty Guacamole
- Lunch: Spinach & Strawberry Meal-Prep Salad
- Dinner: Four-Bean & Pumpkin Chili
- Snack: Air-Fryer Sweet Potato Chips

Day 56

- Breakfast: Fresh Fruit Salad
- Lunch: Chicken with Spinach & Tomato Orzo Salad
- Dinner: Sheet-Pan Chili-Lime Salmon with Potatoes & Peppers
- Snack: Rosemary-Garlic Pecans

Day 57

- Breakfast: Raspberry Overnight Muesli
- Lunch: Mason Jar Power Salad with Chickpeas & Tuna
- Dinner: Chicken & Cucumber Lettuce Wraps with Peanut Sauce
- Snack: Banana & Walnut

Day 58

- Breakfast: Chocolate-Banana Protein Smoothie
- Lunch: Slow-Cooked Ranch Chicken and Vegetables
- Dinner: Peppery Barbecue-Glazed Shrimp with Vegetables & Orzo
- Snack: Avocado-Yogurt Dip

Day 59

- Breakfast: Blueberry Almond Chia Pudding
- Lunch: Lentil Stew with Salsa Verde
- Dinner: Slow-Cooker Chicken & White Bean Stew
- Snack: Apricot-Ginger Energy Balls

Day 60

- Breakfast: White Bean & Avocado Toast
- Lunch: Quinoa Power Salad
- Dinner: Provençal Baked Fish with Roasted Potatoes & Mushrooms
- Snack: Air-Fryer Plantains

About the Author

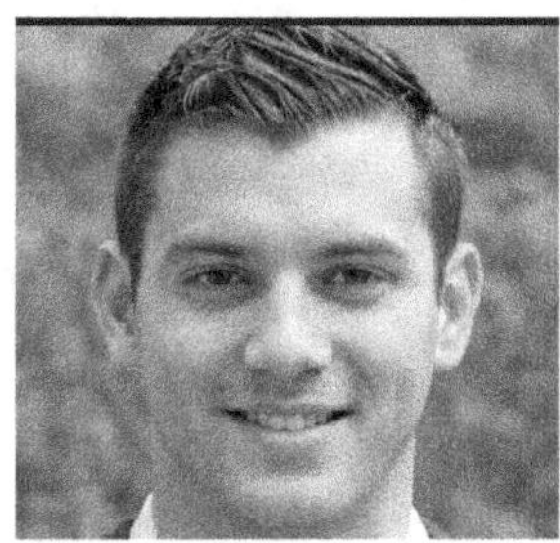 Leopold Knight is a seasoned chef with a passion for transforming ordinary meals into extraordinary, health-conscious experiences. He has a rich culinary background and a commitment to creating recipes that promote overall well-being. Leopold is a culinary artist who specializes in the intersection of delicious and nutritious.

Leopold's culinary journey started in prestigious kitchens, where he honed his skills under the mentorship of distinguished chefs. Fascinated by the complex relationship between food and health, he explored the realms of special diets, developing a unique approach to creating flavorful dishes that contribute to a healthier lifestyle.

With a deep understanding of nutrition and a creative flair for combining wholesome ingredients, Leopold specializes in crafting meals that cater to various dietary preferences and needs. His expertise goes beyond the conventional, embracing a diverse range of special diets that enhance the culinary experience while promoting healthy living.

Outside the kitchen, Leopold Knight is a devoted family man. With a love for shared meals and an understanding of the importance of accommodating diverse tastes and dietary choices, he incorporates his family-centric philosophy into his culinary creations.

Leopold actively shares his culinary philosophy beyond the cookbook, engaging with his audience to impart cooking tips, nutritional insights, and the pure joy of preparing meals that nurture both the body and the spirit.

"DASH Delights" is a testament to Leopold Knight's dedication to merging culinary artistry with health-conscious choices, reflecting his expertise in special diets that make the journey to healthy living a delectable adventure.

Table of Content

Introduction

Overview of the DASH diet

The DASH Diet is a balanced and nutritious way of eating for heart health. The name "DASH" means Dietary Approaches to Stop Hypertension, as it was originally designed to help people with high blood pressure. However, the DASH Diet has also become a general guide for healthy eating, focusing on foods that are rich in nutrients and a good mix of macronutrients.

The main idea of the DASH Diet is to eat more fruits, vegetables, lean proteins, whole grains, and low-fat dairy and to eat less sodium. This way of eating is based on the scientific evidence that our food choices have a significant impact on our overall health. "DASH Delights" is a cookbook that helps you follow these guidelines and also enjoy delicious meals that are not only good for you but also satisfying.

Brief History and Development

The DASH Diet originated from a groundbreaking research by the National Heart, Lung, and Blood Institute (NHLBI) in the early 1990s. The main goal was to find dietary ways to control hypertension, a common health problem affecting millions of people around the world. The DASH study, which was published in 1997, showed how a diet high in fruits, vegetables, and low-fat dairy could lower blood pressure.

Later studies confirmed the effectiveness of the DASH diet and also showed its benefits for other aspects of health. The diet proved to be useful for weight management, overall heart health, and diabetes prevention. The DASH diet became more than just a solution for a specific health issue. It became a way of living that promotes health and wellness.

Importance of a Heart-Healthy Lifestyle

Living a heart-healthy lifestyle is very important in a world where we often neglect our well-being due to the fast pace of life. Heart diseases are still a major cause of death worldwide, which shows the urgent need for preventive actions to protect our heart health. The DASH Diet, which focuses on natural, minimally processed foods, offers a guide to not only lower blood pressure but also live a lifestyle that supports our most essential organ.

The idea that we can enjoy delicious food and take care of our heart health at the same time is the foundation of "DASH Delights." It highlights the fact that living a heart-healthy lifestyle does not mean giving up on pleasure; rather, it means appreciating the variety of flavors that come from wholesome, nutritious foods. As we explore the recipes in the following chapters, keep in mind that each one is a step towards not just a healthier blood pressure but a more fulfilling, tastier life—a life where heart health is not a burden but a joy.

The Science Behind DASH

Principles and Foundation of the DASH Diet

The DASH Diet is based on a set of carefully designed principles. The main idea of DASH is to eat foods that are rich in nutrients and natural, and to eat less sodium and processed foods. The key is to find a balance between important nutrients, especially potassium, calcium, and magnesium.

DASH recommends eating a lot of fruits, vegetables, lean proteins, and whole grains, which all help to provide the nutrition that is essential for heart health. By following these principles, people can start a journey that goes beyond counting calories—it becomes a promise to feed the body with the elements that are needed for optimal function.

Supported Research and Studies

The DASH Diet is not based on stories; it is based on a lot of scientific research. The main DASH study, done by the National Heart, Lung, and Blood Institute (NHLBI) and other institutions, showed how the diet affects blood pressure.This important study, which came out in 1997, showed that people who followed the DASH Diet had lower blood pressure, especially those who had high blood pressure before starting DASH. More research confirmed these results, making DASH a key part of controlling high blood pressure.

Research also shows that the DASH Diet has other benefits for the heart, such as improving cholesterol levels, reducing inflammation, and enhancing heart health. The agreement of the scientific community shows that the DASH Diet is a real way to improve heart health through diet.

As we look at the science behind DASH, we can see that this way of eating is not a trend but a careful plan of nutrients that creates a harmony of health. Based on principles that are backed by science, the DASH Diet helps people to take charge of their heart health through the combination of healthy, nutritious foods.

Explanation of High Blood Pressure

Blood pressure is a measure of how hard the blood pushes against the artery walls. It is important for blood pressure to be balanced for heart health. High blood pressure, or hypertension, means that the blood pressure is too high, which causes stress on the heart and the arteries. This can make the heart work less efficiently and lead to serious health problems.

Blood pressure is expressed by two numbers: systolic pressure (the pressure when the heart pumps) and diastolic pressure (the pressure when the heart relaxes between pumps). A normal blood pressure reading is usually lower than 120/80 mm Hg. Hypertension occurs when these numbers are higher than the normal range, increasing the risk of severe health complications.

Health Risks Associated with Hypertension

High blood pressure, or hypertension, is a serious health problem that can damage the body without causing any symptoms. It affects many organs and systems in the body, not just the heart and blood vessels.

One of the main problems is that high blood pressure can cause atherosclerosis, which is when the arteries become narrow and hard because of plaque buildup. This makes it harder for the blood to flow and can cause clots that can lead to heart attacks and strokes. High blood pressure can also harm the kidneys and reduce their function, which can lead to chronic kidney disease.

Moreover, high blood pressure can affect the eyes and cause vision problems, such as hypertensive retinopathy. It can also affect the brain and increase the risk of cognitive decline and dementia. These health risks show why it is important to take action to control blood pressure effectively.

Benefits of Managing Blood Pressure through Diet

Lifestyle changes, especially diet, are often the first step to managing high blood pressure. Diet can help lower blood pressure and prevent the risks of hypertension without using drugs. Eating a heart-healthy diet has many benefits. First, it helps by eating foods that have potassium, calcium, and magnesium, which can help lower blood pressure. Second, it helps by keeping a healthy weight, which is also important for controlling blood pressure.

The DASH Diet is a good example of a heart-healthy diet. It focuses on natural, nutritious foods and less sodium. It can help lower blood pressure and improve heart health. By changing what we eat, we can take charge of our health and make habits that are good for us in many ways.

Hypertension is not just about numbers; it's about taking action and making choices that are good for our heart. As we follow the way to heart health, we can see how diet can make a difference—small choices that have big effects on our well-being.

How DASH Helps Lower Blood Pressure

The DASH Diet works to lower blood pressure by balancing the nutrients in the food. The most important nutrient is potassium, which can help reduce the high blood pressure caused by sodium. By eating more fruits, vegetables, and low-fat dairy, which have a lot of potassium, DASH helps to create a balance that lowers the effect of too much sodium on the blood vessels.

The DASH Diet also helps by eating less sodium, which is very important for controlling blood pressure. Sodium, which is often found in processed and packaged foods, can make the body hold more water and increase the blood pressure. By choosing foods carefully, DASH tries to create a situation where sodium does not cause high blood pressure.

The diet also helps by eating more whole grains and lean proteins, which can help control blood pressure. Whole grains have fiber and lean proteins make you feel full, which can help with weight management. Weight management is another important factor for regulating blood pressure.

How DASH Supports Weight Management

The DASH Diet, which is known for its good effects on the heart, also helps with losing weight. DASH's basic principles match well with the basics of effective weight management, creating a complete way of eating that goes beyond counting calories.

Importance of Nutrient Density: DASH guides people to eat foods that have a lot of nutrients—such as vitamins, minerals, and other important nutrients—while avoiding processed and high-calorie foods. By eating fruits, vegetables, lean proteins, and whole grains, people can enjoy meals that make them feel good and improve their health.

Feeling Full and Controlling Portions: Many DASH-approved foods have fiber, which makes people feel full and less likely to eat too much. Also, the diet helps people to control their portions wisely, letting them enjoy the tastes of nutritious meals without eating too many calories.

Dealing with Emotional Eating: DASH is more than just a list of dietary rules; it helps people to have a healthy and balanced relationship with food. By eating whole, nourishing foods, people may be less likely to fall into the traps of emotional eating, creating a lasting basis for weight management.

Balancing Calorie Intake and Expenditure

To keep a healthy weight, you need to balance how much you eat and how much you burn. DASH, which focuses on foods that have a lot of nutrients, helps you to do this, giving you a way of eating that goes beyond strict diets.

Being Aware of Calories: DASH doesn't tell you how many calories to eat, but it helps you to be aware of the calories in the foods you eat. By choosing foods that are rich in nutrients and low in calories per gram, you can have meals that make you feel good and don't make you eat too many calories.

The Importance of Macronutrients: DASH understands that you need a balanced amount of macronutrients—proteins, carbohydrates, and fats. This balanced way helps you to have enough energy and avoid the big changes that often happen with fad diets.

Healthy Fats and Weight Management: DASH includes healthy fats, such as those in olive oil, avocados, and nuts, which are good for your heart and also help with weight management. These fats make you feel full, which reduces the chance of eating without thinking.

Physical Activity Recommendations

DASH is mainly about what you eat, but it also knows how important physical activity is for your health and weight. The diet is supported by suggestions for doing regular exercise as part of your routine.

A Balanced Way of Living: DASH helps you to have a balanced way of living that includes eating well and being active. This may include activities like walking, jogging, swimming, or playing sports, depending on what you like and what you can do.

Sticking to It: The focus on sticking to physical activity matches DASH's overall way of thinking about health. You don't lose weight by doing too much exercise but by doing enjoyable, regular activities every day.

Finding What Works for You: DASH understands that physical activity is not the same for everyone. It helps you to find activities that you like, making exercise more fun and helping you to follow a more active way of living.

DASH is a good example of balance—both in what you eat and how you live. By following the ideas of nutrient density, mindful eating, and doing regular physical activity, people who start the DASH journey not only improve their heart health but also create a lasting way of losing weight and being healthy.

Getting Started with DASH

Step-by-Step Guide for Beginners

Starting the DASH journey is more than just changing your diet—it's a change for a better heart health. For beginners, a step-by-step guide can help you to follow the DASH principles in your daily life.

Learn the Basics: Learn about the main ideas of the DASH Diet. This means knowing the key food groups, how to control portions, and why it is important to choose foods that have a lot of nutrients.

Evaluate Your Current Diet: Think about how you eat now. Find areas where you can make DASH-friendly changes. This may include eating less sodium, eating more vegetables, and picking lean protein sources.

Set Realistic Goals: Set goals that you can achieve. Whether it's eating less sodium, eating more fruits and vegetables, or using healthier cooking methods, making realistic goals will help you to change gradually and steadily.

Try DASH Recipes: Try out the many DASH recipes that are available. Try new flavors and combinations to find meals that you like and that follow the DASH principles.

Recommended Daily Servings and Portion Control

The DASH Diet is based on knowing how much of different food groups to eat every day. This helps to get a balanced amount of important nutrients and to control how much you eat.

Fruits and Vegetables: Eat 4–5 servings of fruits and 4–5 servings of vegetables every day. These are colorful, nutritious foods that are very important for DASH nutrition.

Whole Grains: Eat 6–8 servings of whole grains every day. Choose whole wheat, brown rice, quinoa, and oats to get more fiber and feel full.

Lean Proteins: Eat 2 or less servings of lean meats, poultry, or fish every day. You can also try plant-based protein sources like beans, lentils, and tofu.

Dairy: Eat 2 or less servings of low-fat or fat-free dairy products every day. This gives you enough calcium without too much saturated fat.

Nuts, Seeds, and Legumes: Eat 4–5 servings of these healthy foods every week. They have protein, fiber, and good fats that are good for your heart.

Fats and Oils: Keep the total amount of fat you eat within the recommended levels, and focus on healthy fats like those in olive oil, avocados, and nuts.

Grocery Shopping and Meal Planning Tips

The DASH Diet requires smart grocery shopping and meal planning to be successful.

Make a Shopping List: Before going to the store, make a detailed shopping list based on your weekly meal plan. This avoids buying things you don't need and makes sure you have all the ingredients you need.

Buy Fresh Produce: Focus on the fresh produce section, getting fruits and vegetables of different colors. Fresh, whole foods are the main part of DASH nutrition.

Check Labels Carefully: Look at food labels for sodium content, choosing low-sodium or no-salt-added versions when you can. Be aware of hidden sources of sodium in processed foods.

Try Different Protein Sources: Try different kinds of proteins, including lean meats, poultry, fish, and plant-based options. This not only gives you different nutrients but also makes meals more fun.

Plan Balanced Meals: Make a weekly meal plan that includes a variety of food groups. This not only makes your grocery shopping easier but also ensures you have balanced, DASH-friendly meals throughout the week.

Batch Cooking and Meal Prep: Think about batch cooking and meal prepping to make your week easier. Make DASH-friendly meals ahead of time to avoid the temptation of less healthy options when you are busy.

Starting the DASH Diet is not just changing what you eat—it's choosing a lifestyle that puts your heart health first. By following a step-by-step guide, knowing how much to eat, and using smart grocery shopping and meal planning tips, you set the stage for a change that will improve your well-being.

Making DASH-Friendly Choices at Restaurants

Eating out can be hard for those who follow the DASH Diet, but with a smart way of doing it, you can have restaurant meals without hurting your heart.

Look at the Menu and Change It: When you look at the menu, pay attention to dishes that follow DASH ideas. Pick lean protein choices, like grilled chicken or fish, and pick sides with different vegetables. Don't be afraid to change your order—asking for steamed vegetables instead of fries or asking for sauces on the side lets you make your meal fit DASH rules.

Be Smart About How It's Cooked: Think about how it's cooked. Grilled, baked, or steamed dishes are usually healthier than fried or sautéed ones. Also, choosing appetizers as main dishes can help you control how much you eat.

Watch Out for Hidden Sodium: Restaurant meals often have hidden sources of sodium. Ask about how they are prepared, and be careful with sauces and dressings. Asking for them on the side lets you control how much you eat.

Enjoy Yourself Sometimes: While it's important to follow DASH rules, sometimes you can treat yourself. Just be careful with how much you eat and balance higher-calorie choices with healthier ones.

Maintaining DASH Integrity at Social Events

Social events are part of life, and the DASH Diet doesn't have to stop you from having fun. With some planning and awareness, you can go to social events while following DASH rules.

Before the Event: If you can, look at the menu or ask about the dishes they will serve before. This helps you to find DASH-friendly options and plan what you will eat.

Bring DASH-Friendly Food: If you are going to a potluck or bringing food to share, bring something that follows the DASH Diet. A colorful salad, a veggie-based appetizer, or a lean protein dish can be both tasty and DASH-friendly.

Pay Attention to How You Eat: In social settings, it's easy to forget how much you eat and eat more than you need. Pay attention to how you eat by enjoying each bite, noticing when you are hungry and full, and taking your time between servings.

Drink Water or Other Low-Calorie Drinks: Choose water or other drinks that have few calories to stay hydrated. Drink less alcohol, as too much alcohol can make you eat more calories and may make you less aware of what you are eating.

Tell Your Friends and Family About Your Diet: Let your friends and family know about your dietary choices. Having a supportive network can make social situations more enjoyable, and they may even choose restaurants or dishes that suit your DASH goals.

Be Flexible and Adaptable: Social situations are not always perfect, and not every event may follow DASH rules exactly. In such cases, be flexible and make the best choices you can. One bad meal doesn't mean you have failed at your overall dietary efforts.

To go out to eat and socialize while on the DASH Diet, you need a mix of knowledge, mindfulness, and adaptability. By making smart choices at restaurants, planning ahead for social events, and being flexible when needed, you can find a balance between having fun in life's moments and keeping your heart healthy.

Breakfast Recipes

- Spinach & Egg Scramble with Raspberries
- Raspberry Yogurt Cereal Bowl
- Spinach & Egg Tacos
- Overnight Quinoa Pudding
- Raspberry Overnight Muesli
- Homemade Plain Greek Yogurt
- Breakfast Blueberry-Oatmeal Cakes
- Blueberry-Banana Overnight Oats
- Peanut Butter Protein Overnight Oats

Spinach & Egg Scramble with Raspberries

Nutrition Facts || Fat **16g**, Carb **21g**, Protein **18g**, Fiber **7g**, Calories **296**
Prep Time: 10 mins, **Total Time:** 10 mins, **Servings**: 1
Yield: 1 serving

Ingredients

1 teaspoon of canola oil

1 ½ cups (1 ½ ounces) of baby spinach

2 large eggs, lightly beaten

A pinch of kosher salt

A pinch of ground pepper

1 slice of whole-grain bread, toasted

½ cup of fresh raspberries

Directions

In a small nonstick skillet over medium-high heat, heat oil. Stir-fry spinach until wilted, 1 to 2 minutes. Transfer spinach to a plate. Clean the pan, place over medium heat and add eggs. Stir once or twice to cook evenly, until just set, 1 to 2 minutes. Stir in spinach, salt and pepper. Enjoy the scramble with toast and raspberries.

Raspberry Yogurt Cereal Bowl

Nutrition Facts || Fat **5g**, Carb **48g**, Protein **18g**, Fiber **6g**, Calories **290**
Prep Time: 5 mins, **Total Time:** 5 mins, **Servings**: 1
Yield: 1 serving

Ingredients

1 cup of nonfat plain yogurt
½ cup of mini shredded-wheat cereal
¼ cup of fresh raspberries
2 teaspoons of mini chocolate chips
1 teaspoon of pumpkin seeds
¼ teaspoon of ground cinnamon

Directions

Put yogurt in a bowl and sprinkle shredded wheat, raspberries, chocolate chips, pumpkin seeds and cinnamon on top.

Spinach & Egg Tacos

Nutrition Facts || Fat **42g**, Carb **32g**, Protein **21g**, Fiber **8g**, Calories **421**
Active Time: 5 mins, **Total Time**: 5 mins, **Servings**: 1
Yield: 2 Tacos

Ingredients

¼ avocado

1 teaspoon of lime juice

2 hard-boiled eggs, chopped

2 corn of tortillas, warmed

1 cup of chopped spinach, divided

2 tablespoons of shredded Cheddar cheese, divided

2 tablespoons of salsa, divided

Directions

In a small bowl, mash avocado with lime juice and salt. Stir in eggs. Spread the mixture over tortillas and top each one with ½ cup spinach and 1 tablespoon each of cheese and salsa.

Overnight Quinoa Pudding

Nutrition Facts || Fat **9g**, Carb **62g**, Protein **18g**, Fiber **9g**, Calories **394**
Prep Time: 5 mins, **Additional Time**: 8hrs
Total Time: 8 hrs 5 mins, **Servings**: 1
Yield: 1/2 cups

Ingredients

1 cup of cooked and cooled quinoa
¾ cup of plain kefir
1 tablespoon of chia seeds, plus more for serving
2 teaspoons of pure maple syrup
¼ teaspoon of vanilla extract
A dash of ground cinnamon
1 cup of fresh berries for serving

Directions

Mix quinoa, kefir, chia seeds, maple syrup, vanilla and cinnamon in a bowl or jar. Leave it in the fridge overnight. To serve, add berries and more chia, if you like.

Raspberry Overnight Muesli

Nutrition Facts || Fat **8g**, Carb **68g**, Protein **17g**, Fiber **9g**, Calories **401**
Cook Time: 5 mins, **Additional Time**: 7 hrs 55 mins
Total Time: 8 hrs, **Servings**: 1
Yield: 1 serving

Ingredients

¾ cup of nonfat vanilla yogurt

½ cup of old-fashioned rolled oats

½ cup of fresh raspberries

1 tablespoon of toasted chopped almonds

Directions

Mix yogurt and oats in a medium bowl. Cover and leave in the fridge for 8 to 24 hours.

Add raspberries and sprinkle almonds just before eating.

Tips

You can keep in the fridge for up to 24 hours.

Oats that are labeled "gluten-free" should be used by people who have celiac disease or gluten-sensitivity, as wheat and barley often cross-contaminate oats.

Homemade Plain Greek Yogurt

Nutrition Facts || Fat **0g,** Carb **27g**, Protein **18g**, Fiber **0g**, Calories **184**
Active Time: 40 mins, **Additional Time**: 17 hrs 20 mins
Total Time: 18 hrs, **Servings**: 2
Yield: 2 servings

Ingredients

4 cups of nonfat or low-fat milk
¼ cup of nonfat or low-fat plain yogurt

Directions

Heat milk in a large saucepan over medium-high heat, stirring, until it is hot, barely bubbling and reaches 180°F on a thermometer. (Watch it carefully—it can boil over very quickly.)

Carefully pour the hot milk into a clean, heat-safe 5- to 8-cup container. Let it cool, stirring often, until it reaches 110°F. Mix yogurt with ½ cup of the 110°F milk in a small bowl, then stir the mixture back into the warm milk.

Cover the container and wrap it in a clean kitchen towel to help keep it warm. Place it in a very warm place and let it sit, undisturbed, until thick and tangy, at least 8 hours and up to 12 hours. Refrigerate until cold, about 2 hours. The yogurt will thicken a bit more in the refrigerator.

Line a large fine-mesh sieve with 2 layers of cheesecloth and place over a large bowl. Spoon the cooled yogurt into the cheesecloth, then cover and refrigerate for 8 to 24 hours, depending on how thick you want it.

Breakfast Blueberry-Oatmeal Cakes

Nutrition Facts || Fat **9g**, Carb **41g**, Protein **7g**, Fiber **4g**, Calories **264**
Active Time: 15 mins, **Total Time**: 55 mins, **Servings**: 6
Yield: 6

Ingredients

2 ½ cups of old-fashioned rolled oats
1 ½ cups of low-fat milk
1 large egg, lightly beaten
⅓ cup of pure maple syrup
2 tablespoons of canola oil
1 teaspoon of vanilla extract
1 teaspoon of ground cinnamon
1 teaspoon of baking powder
¼ teaspoon of salt
¾ cup of blueberries, fresh or frozen

Directions

Mix oats and milk in a large bowl. Cover and let it soak in the fridge until most of the liquid is absorbed, at least 8 hours and up to 12 hours.

Heat oven to 375℉. Spray a 12-cup nonstick muffin tin with cooking spray.

Add egg, maple syrup, oil, vanilla, cinnamon, baking powder and salt to the soaked oats and stir well. Divide the mixture among the muffin cups (about ¼ cup each). Put 1 tablespoon blueberries on each.

Bake the oatmeal cakes until they bounce back when touched, 25 to 30 minutes. Let them cool in the pan for about 10 minutes. Loosen and remove with a paring knife. Serve warm.

Tips

Wrap tightly and keep in the fridge for up to 2 days or freeze for up to 3 months. To store your food in the freezer for a long time, wrap it in a layer of plastic wrap and then a layer of foil. The plastic will help protect your food from freezer burn while the foil will help prevent off-odors from getting into your food.

Oats that are labeled "gluten-free" should be used by people who have celiac disease or gluten-sensitivity, as wheat and barley often cross-contaminate oats.

Blueberry-Banana Overnight Oats

Nutrition Facts || Fat **6g**, Carb **57g**, Protein **6g**, Fiber **7g**, Calories **285**
Prep Time: 10 mins, **Additional Time**: 5 hrs 50 mins
Total Time: 6 hrs, **Servings**: 1
Yield: 1 cup

Ingredients

½ cup of unsweetened coconut milk beverage

½ cup of old-fashioned oats

½ tablespoon of chia seeds (Optional)

½ banana, mashed

1 teaspoon of maple syrup

A pinch of salt

½ cup of fresh blueberries

1 tablespoon of unsweetened flaked coconut (Optional)

Directions

Mix coconut milk, oats, chia seeds (if using), banana, maple syrup and salt in a jar that holds a pint and stir. Add blueberries and coconut, if you like. Cover and leave in the fridge overnight.

Tips

You can keep in the fridge for up to 1 day.

Oats that are labeled "gluten-free" should be used by people who have celiac disease or gluten-sensitivity, as wheat and barley often cross-contaminate oats.

Peanut Butter Protein Overnight Oats

Nutrition Facts || Fat **9g**, Carb **63g**, Protein **13g**, Fiber **10g**, Calories **368**
Prep Time: 5 mins, **Additional Time**: 7 hrs 55 mins
Total Time: 8 hrs, **Servings**: 1
Yield: 1 cup

Ingredients
½ cup of soymilk or other plant-based milk
½ cup of old-fashioned rolled oats
1 tablespoon of pure maple syrup
1 tablespoon of chia seeds
1 tablespoon of powdered peanut butter
A pinch of salt
½ medium banana, sliced, or ½ cup of berries

Directions
Mix soymilk (or other milk), oats, syrup, chia, powdered peanut butter and salt in a 2-cup mason jar and stir. Leave it in the fridge overnight.

Top with banana or berries and serve.

Tips
After step 1, you can leave in the fridge for up to 4 days.

Oats that are labeled "gluten-free" should be used by people who have celiac disease or gluten-sensitivity, as wheat and barley often cross-contaminate oats.

Lunch Recipes

- Chipotle-Lime Cauliflower Taco Bowls
- Chimichurri Noodle Bowls
- Sweet Potato, Kale & Chicken Salad with Peanut Dressing
- Smoked Salmon Salad Nicoise
- Tomato, Cucumber & White-Bean Salad with Basil Vinaigrette
- White Bean & Veggie Salad
- Lemon-Roasted Vegetable Hummus Bowls
- Mixed Greens with Lentils & Sliced Apple
- Rainbow Grain Bowl with Cashew Tahini Sauce

Chipotle-Lime Cauliflower Taco Bowls

Nutrition Facts || Fat **13g**, Carb **47g**, Protein **13g**, Fiber **12g**, Calories **345**
Prep Time: 20 mins, **Additional Time**: 20 mins
Total Time: 40 mins, **Servings**: 4
Yield: 4 bowls

Ingredients

¼ cup of lime juice (from about 2 limes)
1-2 tablespoons of chopped chipotles in adobo sauce
1 tablespoon of honey
2 cloves of garlic
½ teaspoon of salt
1 small head of cauliflower, cut into bite-size pieces
1 small red onion, halved and thinly sliced
2 cups of cooked quinoa, cooled
1 cup of no-salt-added canned black beans, rinsed
½ cup of crumbled queso fresco
1 cup of shredded red cabbage
1 medium avocado
1 lime, cut into 4 wedges (Optional)

Directions

Heat oven to 450°F. Cover a large baking sheet with foil.

Blend lime juice, chipotles to taste, honey, garlic and salt in a blender. Process until mostly smooth. Put cauliflower in a large bowl; add the sauce and stir to coat. Transfer to the prepared baking sheet. Scatter onion over the cauliflower. Roast, stirring once, until the cauliflower is tender and browned in spots, 18 to 20 minutes; set aside to cool.

Split quinoa among 4 single-serving lidded containers (1/2 cup each). Top each with one-fourth of the cauliflower mixture, ¼ cup black beans and 2 tablespoons cheese. Seal the containers and refrigerate for up to 4 days.

Vent the lid to reheat each container and microwave on High until steaming, up to 2 ½ or 3 minutes. Top with ¼ cup cabbage and ¼ sliced avocado . Serve with a lime wedge, if you like.

Chimichurri Noodle Bowls

Nutrition Facts || Fat **20g**, Carb **28g**, Protein **25g**, Fiber **5g**, Calories **377**
Prep Time: 20 mins, **Total Time**: 20 mins, **Servings**: 4
Yield: 4 noodle bowls

Ingredients
Chimichurri Sauce:
2 cups of fresh flat-leaf parsley
5 cloves of garlic
3 tablespoons of lemon juice
1 tablespoon of fresh oregano or 1 teaspoon of dried
½ teaspoon of crushed red pepper (Optional)
½ teaspoon of salt
¼ teaspoon of ground pepper
½ cup of extra-virgin olive oil

Noodle Bowls:
4 ounces of whole-grain spaghetti
8 cups of zucchini noodles (from 3 medium zucchini)
12 of ounces peeled cooked shrimp
¼ cup of crumbled feta cheese

Directions
Start by boiling a large pot of water for the pasta.

While the water is boiling, make the sauce: Put parsley, garlic, lemon juice, oregano, crushed red pepper (if using), salt and pepper in a food processor and blend until smooth. Slowly pour in oil while the food processor is running. Scrape the sides and blend again until well mixed. Put 2 tablespoons of the sauce in each of 4 small containers with lids and put them in the fridge. Save any extra sauce in the fridge for another use.

To make the noodle bowls: Cook the spaghetti in the boiling water following the package directions. Rinse with cold water, drain, and put in a large bowl; add the zucchini noodles.

Gently mix the spaghetti and zoodles together with tongs or two large forks until well combined. Split among 4 single-serving containers with lids. Add 3 ounces of shrimp and 1 tablespoon of feta cheese to each container.

Close the containers and keep them in the fridge for up to 4 days. Add the chimichurri sauce and toss before eating.

Tips
You can find fresh zucchini noodles in the produce section, or make your own zucchini noodles.

Keep in the fridge for up to 4 days. If you are using precooked frozen shrimp, thaw the shrimp when you are ready to eat.

Sweet Potato, Kale & Chicken Salad with Peanut Dressing

Nutrition Facts || Fat **15g**, Carb **32g**, Protein **30g**, Fiber **6g**, Calories **393**
Prep Time: 15 mins, **Additional Time**: 30 mins
Total Time: 45 mins, **Servings**: 4
Yield: 4 servings

Ingredients

1 pound of sweet potatoes (about 2 medium), scrubbed and cut into 1-inch cubes
1 ½ teaspoons of extra-virgin olive oil
¼ teaspoon of kosher salt
⅛ teaspoon of ground pepper
½ cup of peanut dressing
6 cups of chopped curly kale
2 cups of shredded cooked chicken breast
¼ cup of chopped unsalted peanuts

Directions

Heat the oven to 425 degrees F. Spray a baking sheet with foil and cooking spray lightly. Keep it aside. In a large bowl, mix sweet potatoes with oil, salt and pepper.

Spread the sweet potatoes in one layer on the baking sheet. Bake, flipping once, until they are soft and lightly browned and crispy outside, about 20 minutes. Let them cool before making the bowls.

Put 2 tablespoons of peanut dressing in each of 4 small containers with lids; keep them in the fridge for up to 4 days.

Split kale into 4 single-serving containers (about 1 ½ cups each). Add one-fourth of the roasted sweet potatoes and ½ cup chicken to each container. Close the containers and keep them in the fridge for up to 4 days.

Before eating, pour 1 portion of peanut dressing over each salad and toss well. Sprinkle 1 tablespoon of chopped peanuts on top.

Tips

To make shredded chicken breast, put ¾ pound of boneless, skinless chicken breast in a wide pot and add enough water to cover it. Bring it to a simmer over medium heat. Lower the heat to keep it simmering, cover and cook until the chicken reaches 165 degrees F at the thickest part, 12 to 15 minutes. Take it out and put it on a cutting board. Let it cool a bit, then shred. Let it cool before adding to lunch containers.

Smoked Salmon Salad Niçoise

Nutrition Facts || Fat **6g**, Carb **39g**, Protein **17g**, Fiber **7g**, Calories **271**
Prep Time: 20 mins, **Active Time**: 10 mins
Total Time: 30 mins, **Servings**: 2
Yield: 2 servings

Ingredients

8 ounces of small red potatoes, scrubbed and halved

6 ounces of green beans, preferably thin haricots verts, trimmed and halved

2 tablespoons of reduced-fat mayonnaise

1 tablespoon of white-wine vinegar

1 teaspoon of lemon juice

1 teaspoon of Worcestershire sauce

1 teaspoon of Dijon mustard

½ teaspoon of dried dill

¼ teaspoon of freshly ground pepper

6 cups of mixed salad greens

½ small cucumber, halved, seeded and thinly sliced

12 small cherry or grape tomatoes, halved

4 ounces of smoked salmon, cut into 2-inch pieces

Directions

Get a large bowl of ice water and put it next to the stove. Boil 1 inch of water in a large pot. Put potatoes in a steamer basket over the boiling water, cover and steam until they are soft when you poke them with a fork, 10 to 15 minutes. Use a slotted spoon to move the potatoes to the ice water. Put green beans in the steamer, cover and steam until they are crisp-tender, 4 to 5 minutes. Use a slotted spoon to move the green beans to the ice water. Move the potatoes and beans to a baking sheet with a towel to dry.

While the potatoes and beans are steaming, mix mayonnaise, vinegar, lemon juice, Worcestershire sauce, mustard, dill and pepper in a large bowl. Add the potatoes and green beans, salad greens, cucumber and tomatoes; toss gently to coat.

Split the salad and smoked salmon between 2 plates.

Tomato, Cucumber & White-Bean Salad with Basil Vinaigrette

Nutrition Facts ‖ Fat **15g**, Carb **22g**, Protein **8g**, Fiber **8g**, Calories **246**
Active Time: 25 mins, **Total Time**: 25 mins, **Servings**: 4
Yield: 4 servings

Ingredients

½ cup of packed fresh basil leaves

¼ cup of extra-virgin olive oil

3 tablespoons of red-wine vinegar

1 tablespoon of finely chopped shallot

2 teaspoons of Dijon mustard

1 teaspoon of honey

¼ teaspoon of salt

¼ teaspoon of ground pepper

10 cups of mixed salad greens

1 (15 ounce) can of low-sodium cannellini beans, rinsed

1 cup of halved cherry or grape tomatoes

½ cucumber, halved lengthwise and sliced (1 cup)

Directions

Put basil, oil, vinegar, shallot, mustard, honey, salt and pepper in a small food processor and blend until mostly smooth. Move to a big bowl. Add greens, beans, tomatoes and cucumber. Mix well.

White Bean & Veggie Salad

Nutrition Facts || Fat **25g**, Carb **30g**, Protein **10g**, Fiber **13g**, Calories **360**
Prep Time: 10 mins, **Total Time**: 10 mins, **Servings**: 1
Yield: 4 cups

Ingredients

2 cups of mixed salad greens
¾ cup of veggies of your choice, such as chopped cucumbers and cherry tomatoes
⅓ cup of canned white beans, rinsed and drained
½ avocado, diced
1 tablespoon of red-wine vinegar
2 teaspoons of extra-virgin olive oil
¼ teaspoon of kosher salt
Freshly ground pepper to taste

Directions

Mix greens, veggies, beans and avocado in a medium bowl. Sprinkle with vinegar and oil and season with salt and pepper. Stir well and move to a big plate.

Lemon-Roasted Vegetable Hummus Bowls

Nutrition Facts ‖ Fat **19g**, Carb **40g**, Protein **12g**, Fiber **12g**, Calories **360**
Prep Time: 15 mins, **Additional Time**: 30 mins
Total Time: 45 mins, **Servings**: 4
Yield: 4 servings

Ingredients

1 ½ cups of cauliflower florets
1 ½ cups of broccoli florets
2 cloves of garlic, thinly sliced
1 tablespoon of extra-virgin olive oil
1 teaspoon of dried oregano
¼ teaspoon of salt
¾ cup of diced red bell pepper (1-inch)
¾ cup of diced zucchini (1-inch)
2 teaspoons of lemon zest
2 cups of cooked tricolor quinoa, cooled
1 cup of hummus
4 lemon wedges
1 medium avocado

Directions

Heat the oven to 425 degrees F. Put cauliflower, broccoli and garlic on a baking sheet with edges. Pour oil over them and sprinkle with oregano and salt; toss to coat. Bake for 10 minutes.

Add bell pepper and zucchini to the pan with the vegetables; toss to combine. Bake until the vegetables are tender-crisp and lightly browned, 10 to 15 minutes more. Sprinkle lemon zest over the vegetables; let them cool before making the bowls.

Split the roasted vegetables into 4 single-serving containers. Add ½ cup quinoa and ¼ cup hummus to each container and put a lemon wedge in each container. Close the containers and keep them in the fridge for up to 4 days. When you eat, squeeze the lemon wedge over the bowl and add one-fourth avocado, chopped.

Tips

Keep the containers in the fridge for up to 4 days. Add lemon juice and avocado on top just before eating.

Mixed Greens with Lentils & Sliced Apple

Nutrition Facts ‖ Fat **13g**, Carb **48g**, Protein **13g**, Fiber **14g**, Calories **347**
Prep Time: 10 mins, **Total Time**: 10 mins, **Servings**: 1
Yield: 1 serving

Ingredients

1 ½ cups of mixed salad greens
½ cup of cooked lentils
1 apple, cored and sliced, divided
1 ½ tablespoons of crumbled feta cheese
1 tablespoon of red-wine vinegar
2 teaspoons of extra-virgin olive oil

Directions

Sprinkle lentils, about half of the apple slices and the feta cheese over the greens. Pour vinegar and oil over them. Eat with the rest of the apple slices on the side.

Rainbow Grain Bowl with Cashew Tahini Sauce

Nutrition Facts || Fat **10g**, Carb **54g**, Protein **17g**, Fiber **14g**, Calories **361**
Prep Time: 20 mins, **Total Time:** 20 mins, **Servings:** 1
Yield: 1 bowl

Ingredients

¾ cup of unsalted cashews

½ cup of water

¼ cup of packed parsley leaves

1 tablespoon of lemon juice or cider vinegar

1 tablespoon of extra-virgin olive oil

½ teaspoon of reduced-sodium tamari or soy sauce

¼ teaspoon of salt

½ cup of cooked lentils

½ cup of cooked quinoa

½ cup of shredded red cabbage

¼ cup of grated raw beet

¼ cup of chopped bell pepper

¼ cup of grated carrot

¼ cup of sliced cucumber

1 tablespoon of toasted chopped cashews for garnish

Directions

Mix cashews, water, parsley, lemon juice (or vinegar), oil, tamari (or soy sauce) and salt in a blender until smooth. Put lentils and quinoa in the middle of a flat serving bowl. Add cabbage, beet, pepper, carrot and cucumber on top. Drizzle 2 tablespoons of the cashew sauce over it (keep extra sauce for another use). Sprinkle cashews on top, if you like.

Tips

Soy sauces that are labeled "gluten-free" should be used by people who have celiac disease or gluten-sensitivity, as wheat or other sweeteners and flavors containing gluten may be in soy sauce.

Dinner Recipes

- Slow-Cooker Chicken & White Bean Stew
- Chicken & Cucumber Lettuce Wraps with Peanut Sauce
- Peppery Barbecue-Glazed Shrimp with Vegetables & Orzo
- Cauliflower Fajita Skillet
- Chicken & Sun-Dried Tomato Orzo
- White Turkey Chili
- Stuffed Sweet Potato with Hummus Dressing
- Three-Bean Chili
- Slow-Cooker Chicken & White Bean Stew
- Stuffed Eggplant with Couscous & Almonds
- Spicy Shrimp, Vegetable & Couscous Bowls
- Maple-Roasted Chicken Thighs with Sweet Potato Wedges and Brussels Sprouts
- White Bean Soup with Pasta
- Chicken & Mushroom Ragu
- Baked Halibut with Brussels Sprouts & Quinoa
- Chipotle Chicken Quinoa Burrito Bowl
- Meal-Prep Chili-Lime Chicken Bowls
- Grilled Eggplant & Tomato Pasta
- Stuffed Potatoes with Salsa & Beans
- One-Pan Chicken & Asparagus Bake

Slow-Cooker Chicken & White Bean Stew

Nutrition Facts || Fat **11g**, Carb **54g**, Protein **44g**, Fiber **27g**, Calories **493**
Prep Time: 15 mins, **Additional Time:** 7 hrs 20 mins
Total Time: 7 hrs 45 mins, **Servings**: 6
Yield: 7 ½ cups

Ingredients

1 pound of dried cannellini beans, soaked overnight and drained
6 cups of unsalted chicken broth
1 cup of chopped yellow onion
1 cup of sliced carrots
1 teaspoon of finely chopped fresh rosemary
1 (4 ounce) of Parmesan cheese rind plus 2/3 cup of grated Parmesan, divided
2 bone-in chicken breasts (1 pound each)
4 cups of chopped kale
1 tablespoon of lemon juice
½ teaspoon of kosher salt
½ teaspoon of ground pepper
2 tablespoons of extra-virgin olive oil
¼ cup of flat-leaf parsley leaves

Directions

Put beans, broth, onion, carrots, rosemary and Parmesan rind in a slow cooker that can hold 6 quarts. Add chicken on top. Cover and cook on Low until the beans and vegetables are soft, 7 to 8 hours.

Take the chicken out and put it on a clean cutting board; let it cool a bit, about 10 minutes. Pull the chicken apart, throwing away bones.Put the chicken back in the slow cooker and add kale. Cover and cook on High until the kale is soft, 20 to 30 minutes.

Add lemon juice, salt and pepper; throw away the Parmesan rind. Serve the stew with oil drizzled over it and Parmesan and parsley sprinkled on top.

Chicken & Cucumber Lettuce Wraps with Peanut Sauce

Nutrition Facts || Fat **26g**, Carb **44g**, Protein **34g**, Fiber **11g**, Calories **521**
Prep Time: 40 mins, **Total Time**: 40 mins, **Servings**: 4
Yield: 8 lettuce wraps

Ingredients

¼ cup of creamy peanut butter

2 tablespoons of low-sodium soy sauce

2 tablespoons of honey

2 tablespoons of water

2 teaspoons of toasted sesame oil

2 teaspoons of olive oil

3 scallions, sliced, white and green parts separated

1 serrano pepper, seeded and minced (2 tsp.)

1 tablespoon of minced fresh ginger

2 teaspoons of minced fresh garlic

1 pound of ground chicken breast

1 cup of diced jicama

16 Bibb of lettuce leaves

1 cup of cooked brown rice

1 cup of halved and thinly sliced English cucumber

½ cup of fresh cilantro leaves

Lime wedges, for serving

Directions

Mix peanut butter, soy sauce, honey, water, and sesame oil in a small bowl.

Warm olive oil in a big nonstick skillet over medium heat. Add scallion whites, serrano, ginger, and garlic; cook until they begin to soften, about 2 minutes. Add chicken; cook, smashing it with a spoon or potato masher, until done, 3 to 4 minutes.

Pour the peanut sauce over the chicken mixture; cook until the sauce gets thicker, about 3 minutes. Take it off the heat. Stir in jicama and scallion greens.

To eat, make 8 piles of 2 lettuce leaves each. Split rice, the chicken mixture, cucumber, and cilantro among the lettuce cups. Eat with lime wedges.

Peppery Barbecue-Glazed Shrimp with Vegetables & Orzo

Nutrition Facts || Fat **9g**, Carb **41g**, Protein **30g**, Fiber **10g**, Calories **360**
Prep Time: 30 mins, **Total Time**: 30 mins, **Servings**: 4
Yield: 8 cups

Ingredients

1 pound of peeled and deveined jumbo shrimp, thawed if frozen
1 teaspoon of paprika
½ teaspoon of garlic powder
½ teaspoon of dried oregano, crushed
¼ teaspoon of ground pepper
⅛ teaspoon of cayenne pepper
1 cup of whole-grain orzo
3 scallions
2 tablespoons of olive oil, divided
2 cups of coarsely chopped zucchini
1 cup of coarsely chopped bell pepper
½ cup of thinly sliced celery
1 cup of cherry tomatoes, halved
½ teaspoon of salt
2 tablespoons of barbecue sauce
Lemon wedges, for serving

Directions

Put shrimp in a medium bowl. Mix paprika, garlic powder, oregano, pepper and cayenne in a small bowl. Sprinkle the spice mix over the shrimp; toss to coat and keep aside.

Boil a large pot of water. Cook orzo as per package directions; drain. Put it back in the hot pot; cover and keep warm.

While the orzo is cooking, cut scallions, separating white and green parts. Warm 1 tablespoon oil in a medium skillet over medium-high heat. Add the scallion whites, zucchini, bell pepper and celery; cook, stirring sometimes, until the vegetables are tender-crisp, about 5 minutes. Add tomatoes; cook until soft, 2 to 3 minutes more. Add the vegetables to the pot with the orzo. Add salt; stir to combine.

In the same skillet, warm the remaining 1 tablespoon oil over medium heat. Add the shrimp; cook, turning once, until they are not clear, 4 to 6 minutes. Pour barbecue sauce over them. Cook and stir until the shrimp are covered, about 1 minute.

Serve the shrimp with the vegetable mix. Sprinkle scallion greens on top and serve with lemon wedges, if you like.

Tips
Frozen shrimp can thaw quickly. Put frozen shrimp in a big bowl with ice water. Let it stand for 20 minutes.

Cauliflower Fajita Skillet

Nutrition Facts ‖ Fat **11g**, Carb **48g**, Protein **9g**, Fiber **9g**, Calories **302**
Active Time: 15 mins, **Total Time:** 45 mins, **Servings**: 6
Yield: 6 servings

Ingredients

1 medium head of cauliflower, trimmed and thinly sliced
1 medium red bell pepper, sliced
1 medium onion, sliced
3 tablespoons of extra-virgin olive oil
1 ½ teaspoons of chili powder
1 teaspoon of ground cumin
½ teaspoon of ground coriander
½ teaspoon of salt
¼ teaspoon of ground pepper
½ cup of pico de gallo
¼ cup of chopped pickled jalapeño peppers
Chopped fresh cilantro for garnish
1 14-ounce can of light-in-sodium refried beans, warmed
12 corn of tortillas, warmed

Directions

Put a rack in the top part of the oven and a big cast-iron skillet on it. Heat to 425°F.

Mix cauliflower, bell pepper, onion and oil in a medium bowl and toss to coat. Add chili powder, cumin, coriander, salt and pepper and toss until well coated. Carefully put the mix in the hot pan. Roast, stirring once, until the vegetables are soft, about 30 minutes.

Set the broiler to high. Broil the vegetables until lightly browned for about 2 minutes. Sprinkle pico de gallo, jalapeños and cilantro over the vegetables, if you want. Eat with refried beans and tortillas.

Chicken & Sun-Dried Tomato Orzo

Nutrition Facts || Fat **12g**, Carb **54g**, Protein **36g**, Fiber **10g**, Calories **456**
Cook Time: 30 mins, **Total Time**: 30 mins, **Servings**: 4
Yield: 12 to 4 oz. chicken & cups pasta

Ingredients

8 ounces of orzo, preferably whole-wheat

1 cup of water

½ cup of chopped sun-dried tomatoes, (not oil-packed), divided

1 plum of tomato, diced

1 clove of garlic, peeled

3 teaspoons of chopped fresh marjoram, divided

1 tablespoon of red-wine vinegar

2 teaspoons plus 1 tablespoon of extra-virgin olive oil, divided

4 boneless, skinless chicken breasts, trimmed (1-1 ¼ pounds)

¼ teaspoon of salt

¼ teaspoon of freshly ground pepper

1 9-ounce package of frozen artichoke hearts, thawed

½ cup of finely shredded Romano cheese, divided

Directions

Boil orzo in a big pot of water until it is just soft, 8 to 10 minutes or as per package directions. Drain and rinse.

While the orzo is cooking, put 1 cup water, ¼ cup sun-dried tomatoes, plum tomato, garlic, 2 teaspoons marjoram, vinegar and 2 teaspoons oil in a blender. Blend until there are only a few chunks left.

Sprinkle salt and pepper on both sides of the chicken. Warm the remaining 1 tablespoon oil in a large skillet over medium-high heat. Add the chicken and cook, adjusting the heat as needed to avoid burning, until golden outside and not pink inside, 3 to 5 minutes per side. Take it out and put it on a plate; cover with foil to keep it warm.

Put the tomato sauce in the pan and bring it to a boil. Take out ½ cup sauce to a small bowl. Add the rest ¼ cup sun-dried tomatoes to the pan with the orzo, artichoke hearts and 6 tablespoons cheese. Cook, stirring, until hot, 1 to 2 minutes. Split into 4 plates.

Cut the chicken. Put sliced chicken on each plate of pasta with 2 tablespoons of the saved tomato sauce and some of the remaining cheese and marjoram.

White Turkey Chili

Nutrition Facts ‖ Fat **14g**, Carb **38g**, Protein **28g**, Fiber **10g**, Calories **350**
Cook Time: 40 mins, **Additional Time**: 50 mins
Total Time: 1 hrs 30 mins, **Servings**: 6
Yield: 6 servings

Ingredients

3 tablespoons of extra-virgin olive oil or canola oil

1 pound of 93%-lean ground turkey

1 large onion, diced

4 cloves of garlic, minced

2 medium zucchini, diced (about 3 ½ cups)

½ cup of bulgur

2 tablespoons of dried oregano

4 teaspoons of ground cumin

½ teaspoon of ground coriander

½ teaspoon of white pepper

¼ teaspoon of salt

2 15-ounce cans of no-salt-added white beans, rinsed

2 4-ounce cans of green chiles, mild or hot

4 cups of reduced-sodium chicken broth

Directions

Warm oil in a Dutch oven over medium-high heat. Add turkey, onion and garlic. Cook, breaking up the meat with a wooden spoon, until the meat is cooked through, 3 to 5 minutes.

Add zucchini and cook, stirring now and then, until the zucchini is beginning to soften, 5 to 7 minutes.

Add bulgur, oregano, cumin, coriander, white pepper and salt and cook, stirring, until fragrant, 30 seconds to 1 minute.

Mix in white beans and chiles, then pour in broth; bring to a boil.Lower the heat to a simmer, partly cover the pot and cook, stirring sometimes, until the liquid is reduced and thickened and the bulgur is soft, about 50 minutes.

Tips

Cover and keep in the fridge for up to 3 days or freeze for up to 3 months.

Stuffed Sweet Potato with Hummus Dressing

Nutrition Facts ‖ Fat **7g**, Carb **85g**, Protein **21g**, Fiber **22g**, Calories **472**
Prep Time: 15 mins, **Additional Time**: 5 mins
Total Time: 20 mins, **Servings**: 1
Yield: 1 potato

Ingredients

1 large sweet potato, scrubbed
¾ cup of chopped kale
1 cup of canned black beans, rinsed
¼ cup of hummus
2 tablespoons of water

Directions

Poke holes all over the sweet potato with a fork. Cook it in the microwave on High until it is soft, 7 to 10 minutes.

While the sweet potato is cooking, rinse kale and drain, leaving some water on the leaves. Put it in a medium saucepan; cover and cook over medium-high heat, stirring once or twice, until it is wilted. Add beans; add a tablespoon or two of water if the pot is dry. Keep cooking, uncovered, stirring now and then, until the mix is hot, 1 to 2 minutes.

Cut the sweet potato open and put the kale and bean mix on top. Mix hummus and 2 tablespoons water in a small dish. Add more water as needed to get the desired consistency. Pour the hummus dressing over the stuffed sweet potato.

Three-Bean Chili

Nutrition Facts || Fat **8g**, Carb **48g**, Protein **26g**, Fiber **15g**, Calories **358**
Cook Time: 45 mins, **Additional Time**: 2 hrs 45 mins
Total Time: 3 hrs 30 mins, **Servings**: 8
Yield: 8 servings

Ingredients

2 tablespoons of cumin seeds

2 tablespoons of chili powder

1 tablespoon of paprika

2 teaspoons of dried oregano, preferably Mexican

½ teaspoon of cayenne pepper

3 teaspoons of canola oil, divided

1 pound of beef round, trimmed, cut into ½-inch chunks

3 onions, chopped

1 green bell pepper, seeded and chopped

6 cloves of garlic, finely chopped (2 tablespoons)

2 jalapeño peppers, seeded and finely chopped

8 sun-dried tomatoes, (not packed in oil), snipped into small pieces

2 dried ancho chiles, seeds & stems removed, snipped into thin strips (optional)

12 ounces of dark beer, such as porter or stout

1 28-ounce can of plum tomatoes, with juices

1 tablespoon of grated unsweetened chocolate

1 teaspoon of sugar, or honey to taste

2 bay leaves

2 cups of water

1 19-ounce can of kidney beans, rinsed

1 19-ounce can of white beans, such as Great Northern, rinsed

1 19-ounce can of black beans, rinsed

¼ cup of chopped fresh cilantro, (optional)

2 tablespoons of lime juice
Salt & freshly ground pepper, to taste
Nonfat plain yogurt, chopped scallion greens and shredded sharp Cheddar cheese, for garnish

Directions

In a small dry skillet over medium heat, toast cumin seeds, stirring, until they smell good, 1 to 2 minutes. Crush them to a fine powder in a mortar and pestle or spice grinder. Put them in a small bowl; add chili powder, paprika, oregano and cayenne. Mix well; keep aside.

Warm 1 ½ teaspoons of the oil in a big heavy pot over high heat. Add beef, in parts if needed, and cook until browned on all sides, about 3 minutes. Take it out and put it on a plate with paper towels and keep aside.

Lower the heat to medium and add the remaining 1 ½ teaspoons oil to the pan. Add onions and bell pepper. Cook, stirring, until the onions are soft and golden brown, 7 to 10 minutes. Add garlic, jalapeños, sun-dried tomatoes, anchos chiles (if using), and the spice mix you made. Stir until it smells good, about 2 minutes. Add beer, bring to a simmer and cook for 10 minutes, scraping up any brown bits stuck to the bottom of the pan. Add tomatoes and their juices, chocolate, sugar, bay leaves and the beef you browned. Add water and bring to a simmer. Cover the pot and simmer, stirring sometimes, until the beef is very soft, 1 ½ to 2 hours.

Add kidney beans, white beans and black beans and cook until the chili is thick, 30 to 45 minutes more. Take out the bay leaves. Stir in cilantro, if using, and lime juice; season with salt and pepper as you like. Serve with toppings.

Tips

Cover and keep in the fridge for up to 2 days or freeze for up to 6 weeks.

Ancho chiles are dried poblano peppers. They are one of the most popular dried chiles used in Mexico. They have a mild, sweet, spicy flavor. You can find ground ancho chile with other spices in big supermarkets, or use ground chili powder with a pinch of cayenne.

Slow-Cooker Chicken & White Bean Stew

Nutrition Facts || Fat **11g**, Carb **54g**, Protein **44g**, Fiber **27g**, Calories **493**
Prep Time: 15 mins, **Active Time**: 10 mins, **Additional Time**: 7 hrs 20 mins
Total Time: 7 hrs 45 mins, **Servings**: 6
Yield: 7 ½ cups

Ingredients

1 pound of dried cannellini beans, soaked overnight and drained
6 cups of unsalted chicken broth
1 cup of chopped yellow onion
1 cup of sliced carrots
1 teaspoon of finely chopped fresh rosemary
1 (4 ounce) of Parmesan cheese rind plus 2/3 cup of grated Parmesan, divided
2 bone-in chicken breasts (1 pound each)
4 cups of chopped kale
1 tablespoon of lemon juice
½ teaspoon of kosher salt
½ teaspoon of ground pepper
2 tablespoons of extra-virgin olive oil
¼ cup of flat-leaf parsley leaves

Directions

Put beans, broth, onion, carrots, rosemary and Parmesan rind in a slow cooker that can hold 6 quarts. Add chicken on top. Cover and cook on Low until the beans and vegetables are soft, 7 to 8 hours.

Take the chicken out and put it on a clean cutting board; let it cool a bit, about 10 minutes. Pull the chicken apart, throwing away bones.

Put the chicken back in the slow cooker and add kale. Cover and cook on High until the kale is soft, 20 to 30 minutes.

Add lemon juice, salt and pepper; throw away the Parmesan rind. Serve the stew with oil drizzled over it and Parmesan and parsley sprinkled on top.

Stuffed Eggplant with Couscous & Almonds

Nutrition Facts || Fat **33g**, Carb **35g**, Protein **9g**, Fiber **11g**, Calories **457**
Prep Time: 30 mins, **Total Time**: 30 mins, **Servings**: 4
Yield: 4 servings

Ingredients

⅔ cup of water plus 1 tablespoon, divided
½ cup of whole-wheat couscous
½ teaspoon of salt, divided
2 medium eggplants (about 1 pound each)
3 tablespoons of extra-virgin olive oil, divided
¼ teaspoon of ground pepper
1 clove of garlic, finely chopped
⅓ cup of mayonnaise
2 teaspoons of harissa paste or ½ teaspoon of harissa seasoning
½ cup of chopped smoke-flavored almonds
½ cup of chopped fresh parsley

Directions

Heat the grill to medium-high.

In a small saucepan, bring 2/3 cup water, couscous and 1/8 teaspoon salt to a boil over high heat. Take it off the heat, cover and keep aside.

Cut the eggplants in half through the stem; brush the cut sides with 2 tablespoons oil and sprinkle with ¼ teaspoon salt and pepper. Grill the eggplants, turning once halfway, until they are charred and soft, 10 to 12 minutes. Let them cool for 5 minutes.

While the eggplants are cooling, make a paste with garlic and the remaining 1/8 teaspoon salt on a cutting board with a fork. In a small bowl, mix the garlic paste, mayonnaise, harissa and the remaining 1 tablespoon water.

Carefully scoop out the eggplant flesh and chop it, leaving a ¼-inch-thick wall. Stir the eggplant flesh into the couscous with almonds, parsley and the remaining 1 tablespoon oil. Fill the eggplant shells with the couscous mixture. Serve with the sauce.

Tips
Whole-wheat couscous is made by rolling coarse semolina flour, resulting in small round granules. It has three times more fiber than white couscous.

Spicy Shrimp, Vegetable & Couscous Bowls

Nutrition Facts || Fat **18g**, Carb **52g**, Protein **28g**, Fiber **6g**, Calories **478**
Active Time: 20 mins, **Total Time**: 20 mins, **Servings**: 4
Yield: 4 servings

Ingredients

1 ½ cups of whole-wheat pearl couscous

1 small red bell pepper, chopped

½ cup of snow peas, trimmed and sliced

3 tablespoons of sliced fresh basil, divided

3 tablespoons of sliced fresh mint, divided

1 cup of chopped fresh cilantro

2 tablespoons of lime juice

1 tablespoon of rice vinegar

1 tablespoon of water

1 ½ teaspoons of sambal oelek

1 ½ teaspoons of grated fresh ginger

1 large clove of garlic, crushed and peeled

½ teaspoon of ground pepper, divided

⅛ teaspoon of salt

5 tablespoons of grapeseed oil, divided

1 pound of large raw shrimp (16-20 count), peeled and deveined

Directions

Boil couscous as per package directions. Drain, rinse and put in a big bowl. Add bell pepper, snow peas and 2 tablespoons each of basil and mint.

While the couscous is cooking, put cilantro, lime juice, vinegar, water, sambal oelek, ginger, garlic, ¼ teaspoon pepper and salt in a blender. Blend until smooth. Slowly pour in 4 tablespoons oil while the blender is running. Keep aside 2 tablespoons of the dressing. Mix the rest of the dressing with the couscous and vegetables.

Warm the remaining 1 tablespoon oil in a large skillet over high heat. Dry the shrimp and sprinkle with the remaining ¼ teaspoon pepper. Put them in the pan and cook, turning once, until they are done, about 2 minutes per side. Eat the shrimp and couscous mix with the 2 tablespoons dressing you saved and the remaining 1 tablespoon each of basil and mint.

Tip

Sambal oelek is a thick Indonesian sauce made with chiles, vinegar and salt that adds a spicy kick to the dressing here. You can find it in grocery stores or Asian grocery stores. Use the rest of it in stir-fries, noodle dishes or instead of your favorite hot sauce.

Maple-Roasted Chicken Thighs with Sweet Potato Wedges and Brussels Sprouts

Nutrition Facts || Fat **14g**, Carb **45g**, Protein **34g**, Fiber **9g**, Calories **436**
Prep Time: 20 mins, **Additional Time**: 30 mins
Total Time: 50 mins, **Servings**: 4
Yield: 4 servings

Ingredients

2 tablespoons of pure maple syrup

4 teaspoons of olive oil

1 tablespoon of snipped fresh thyme

½ teaspoon of salt

½ teaspoon of black pepper

1 pound of sweet potatoes, peeled and cut into 1-inch wedges

1 pound of Brussels sprouts, trimmed and halved

Nonstick cooking spray

4 bone-in chicken thighs, skinned

3 tablespoons of snipped dried cranberries

3 tablespoons of chopped pecans, toasted

Directions

Heat the oven to 425 degrees F.

Mix maple syrup, 1 tsp. of the oil, the thyme, ¼ tsp. of the salt, and ¼ tsp. of the pepper in a small bowl. In a big bowl, toss sweet potatoes and Brussels sprouts with the remaining 1 tbsp. oil and ¼ tsp. each of salt and pepper.

Cover a 15x10-inch baking pan with foil. Heat the pan in the oven for 5 minutes. Take the pan out of the oven and spray with cooking spray.

Put chicken, skin sides down, in the middle of the pan. Put vegetables around the chicken. Bake 15 minutes. Turn chicken and vegetables over; brush with maple syrup mix. Bake 15 minutes more or until chicken is done (at least 175 degrees F) and potatoes are soft. Sprinkle with pecans and cranberries and serve.

White Bean Soup with Pasta

Nutrition Facts || Fat **5g**, Carb **49g**, Protein **12g**, Fiber **9g**, Calories **277**
Active Time: 15 mins, **Total Time**: 25 mins, **Servings**: 6
Yield: 6 servings

Ingredients

1 tablespoon of extra-virgin olive oil

1 ½ cups of frozen mirepoix (diced onion, celery and carrot)

2 cloves of garlic, minced

1 teaspoon of Italian seasoning

1 teaspoon of salt

¼ teaspoon of crushed red pepper

¼ teaspoon of ground pepper

1 28-ounce can of no-salt-added diced tomatoes

2 cups of low-sodium no-chicken broth or chicken broth

1 15-ounce can of low-sodium cannellini beans, rinsed

8 ounces of small whole-wheat pasta, such as elbows

1 ½ cups of frozen cut-leaf spinach

4 tablespoons of grated Parmesan cheese

Directions

Boil a big pot of water. Warm oil in a big pot over medium-high heat. Add mirepoix and cook, stirring, until soft, about 3 minutes. Add garlic, Italian seasoning, salt, crushed red pepper and black pepper and cook, stirring, until it smells good, about 1 minute. Add tomatoes and their juices, broth and beans and bring to a boil. Lower the heat to keep it simmering. Cover and cook, stirring sometimes, until the tomatoes start to break down, about 10 minutes.

While the soup is cooking, cook pasta in the boiling water for 1 minute less than the package directions. Drain.

Mix spinach into the soup. Mix in the pasta just before eating. Serve with Parmesan on top.

Chicken & Mushroom Ragu

Nutrition Facts || Fat **17g**, Carb **51g**, Protein **28g**, Fiber **8g**, Calories **464**
Active Time: 30 mins, **Total Time:** 40 mins, **Servings**: 8
Yield: 8 servings

Ingredients

1 28-ounce can of no-salt whole peeled tomatoes, preferably San Marzano
¼ cup of extra-virgin olive oil
1 medium onion, chopped
2 medium carrots, chopped
8 ounces of cremini mushrooms, quartered
1 ¾ pounds of boneless, skinless chicken thighs, trimmed, cut into 1-inch pieces
2 cloves of garlic, grated
¼ cup of tomato paste
½ cup of dry red wine
½ teaspoon of salt
¼ teaspoon of crushed red pepper
1 tablespoon of chopped fresh rosemary
1 pound of whole-wheat linguine or fettuccine
½ cup of grated Romano cheese
½ cup of chopped fresh parsley

Directions

Boil a big pot of water.

Squeeze tomatoes and their juice in a medium bowl. Break the tomatoes into pieces with your hands.

Warm oil in an electric pressure cooker on Sauté mode. Add onion, carrots and mushrooms; cook, stirring, until the mushrooms give out their liquid, about 5 minutes. Add chicken, garlic and tomato paste. Cook, stirring sometimes, until the chicken is covered and the mix at the bottom of the pan is starting to brown, about 4 minutes. Add wine, salt, crushed red pepper and the tomatoes. Cook, scraping up the browned bits, until it starts to boil, about 2 minutes. Turn off the heat.

Lock and close the lid. For 10 minutes, cook at High pressure. Release the pressure by hand. Stir in rosemary.

While the sauce is cooking, cook pasta as per package directions. Drain and serve with the sauce, cheese and parsley on top.

Tips
Keep the sauce (Steps 2-4) in the fridge for up to 3 days or freeze for up to 3 months.

Baked Halibut with Brussels Sprouts & Quinoa

Nutrition Facts || Fat **17g**, Carb **36g**, Protein **30g**, Fiber **8g**, Calories **406**
Prep Time: 15 mins, **Additional Time**: 15 mins
Total Time: 30 mins, **Servings**: 4
Yield: 4 servings

Ingredients

1 pound of Brussels sprouts, trimmed and sliced
1 fennel bulb, trimmed and cut into strips
1 tablespoon plus 1 teaspoon of olive oil, divided
½ teaspoon of salt, divided
½ teaspoon of ground pepper, divided
1 (1 pound) of halibut fillet, cut into 4 portions
4 cloves of garlic, minced, divided
3 tablespoons of lemon juice
2 tablespoons of unsalted butter, melted
2 cups of cooked quinoa
¼ cup of chopped sun-dried tomatoes
¼ cup of chopped pitted Kalamata olives
2 tablespoons of chopped fresh Italian parsley or fennel fronds

Directions

Put racks in the top and bottom thirds of the oven; heat to 400 degrees F.

Mix Brussels sprouts, fennel, 1 Tbsp. oil, and ¼ tsp. each salt and pepper in a big bowl; toss to coat. Put them in one layer on a big baking sheet with edges. Bake, stirring sometimes, until soft, 20 to 25 minutes.

While the vegetables are baking, put halibut on another big baking sheet with edges and sprinkle with half of the garlic and the remaining ¼ tsp. each salt and pepper. Mix lemon juice and melted butter in a small bowl. Pour or brush half of it over the fish. Bake until the fish is not clear and breaks easily with a fork, 12 to 15 minutes.

While the fish is baking, mix quinoa, the remaining 1 tsp. oil, sun-dried tomatoes, olives, and parsley (or fennel fronds) in a medium bowl.

Add the remaining garlic to the lemon-butter mix. Drizzle it over the vegetables and bake for 1 minute more. Eat the halibut and vegetables with the quinoa mix.

Chipotle Chicken Quinoa Burrito Bowl

Nutrition Facts ‖ Fat **19g**, Carb **36g**, Protein **36g**, Fiber **9g**, Calories **452**
Active Time: 30 mins, **Total Time**: 30 mins, **Servings**: 4
Yield: 4 burrito bowls

Ingredients
1 tablespoon of finely chopped chipotle peppers in adobo sauce
1 tablespoon of extra-virgin olive oil
½ teaspoon of garlic powder
½ teaspoon of ground cumin
1 pound of boneless, skinless chicken breast
¼ teaspoon of salt
2 cups of cooked quinoa
2 cups of shredded romaine lettuce
1 cup of canned pinto beans, rinsed
1 ripe avocado, diced
¼ cup of prepared pico de gallo or other salsa
¼ cup of shredded Cheddar or Monterey Jack cheese
Lime wedges, for serving

Directions
Heat the grill to medium-high or heat the broiler. Mix chipotles, oil, garlic powder and cumin in a small bowl.

Brush the grill rack or a baking sheet with edges, if broiling. Sprinkle salt on the chicken. Grill the chicken for 5 minutes or broil it on the baking sheet for 9 minutes. Turn, brush with the chipotle sauce and keep cooking until a thermometer put in the thickest part shows 165 degrees F, 3 to 5 minutes more on the grill or 9 minutes more under the broiler. Take it out and put it on a clean cutting board. Cut into small pieces.

Make each burrito bowl with ½ cup quinoa, ½ cup chicken, ½ cup lettuce, ¼ cup beans, ¼ avocado, 1 tablespoon pico de gallo (or other salsa) and 1 tablespoon cheese. Eat with a lime wedge.

Tips

To brush a grill rack, brush a folded paper towel with oil, hold it with tongs and rub it over the rack. Do not spray a hot grill with cooking spray.

Meal-Prep Chili-Lime Chicken Bowls

Nutrition Facts || Fat **14g**, Carb **47g**, Protein **29g**, Fiber **9g**, Calories **413**
Prep Time: 25 mins, **Additional Time**: 5 mins
Total Time: 30 mins, **Servings**: 4
Yield: 8 cups

Ingredients

1 cup of cooked quinoa
1 cup of cooked brown rice
1 pound of cooked Chili-Lime Chicken
1 cup of julienned jicama
1 cup of frozen corn, thawed
1 cup of pico de gallo
1 avocado, diced
½ cup of chopped fresh cilantro
Lime wedges
Hot sauce, such as Cholula

Directions

Mix quinoa and rice together and put them in 4 separate containers that have lids. Add chicken, jicama, corn, pico de gallo and cilantro on top of each container, distributing them equally. Close the lids and keep the containers in the fridge for up to 4 days. Enjoy with avocado pieces, lime slices and hot sauce.

Tips

Store the containers with lids in the fridge for up to 4 days.

Grilled Eggplant & Tomato Pasta

Nutrition Facts || Fat **19g**, Carb **62g**, Protein **14g**, Fiber **12g**, Calories **449**
Active Time: 30 mins, **Total Time**: 30 mins, **Servings**: 4
Yield: 4 servings

Ingredients

1 pound of plum tomatoes, chopped

4 tablespoons of extra-virgin olive oil, divided

2 teaspoons of chopped fresh oregano

1 clove of garlic, grated

½ teaspoon of ground pepper

¼ teaspoon of crushed red pepper

½ teaspoon of salt

1 ½ pounds of eggplant, cut into ½-inch-thick slices

½ cup of chopped fresh basil

8 ounces of whole-wheat penne

¼ cup of shaved ricotta salata or crumbled feta cheese

Directions

Set a big pot of water to boil. Heat up the grill to medium-high.

In a big bowl, toss the tomatoes with 3 tablespoons of oil, oregano, garlic, pepper, crushed red pepper and salt.

Brush the remaining 1 tablespoon of oil on the eggplant. Grill them, flipping once, until they are soft and have some char marks, about 4 minutes for each side. Let them cool down for 10 minutes. Cut them into small pieces and add them to the tomatoes along with the basil.

While that's happening, cook the pasta following the directions on the package. Drain it.

Put the tomato mixture over the pasta. Sprinkle some cheese on top.

Stuffed Potatoes with Salsa & Beans

Nutrition Facts || Fat **8g**, Carb **57g**, Protein **9g**, Fiber **11g**, Calories **324**
Prep Time: 10 mins, **Additional Time**: 15 mins
Total Time: 25 mins, **Servings**: 4
Yield: 4 potatoes

Ingredients

4 medium russet potatoes
½ cup of fresh salsa
1 ripe avocado, sliced
1 (15 ounce) can of pinto beans, rinsed, warmed and lightly mashed
4 teaspoons of chopped pickled jalapeños

Directions

Make holes all over the potatoes with a fork. Microwave them on Medium, flipping them once or twice, until they are soft, about 20 minutes. (Or, you can bake the potatoes in the oven at 425 degrees F until they are done, 45 minutes to 1 hour.) Move them to a clean cutting board and let them cool a bit.

Use a kitchen towel to hold them and cut them lengthwise to open them, but don't cut through. Squeeze the ends to show the inside.

Put some salsa, avocado, beans and jalapeños on each potato. Eat them while they are hot.

One-Pan Chicken & Asparagus Bake

Nutrition Facts || Fat **14g**, Carb **31g**, Protein **28g**, Fiber **6g**, Calories **352**
Prep Time: 15 mins, **Additional Time:** 20 mins
Total Time: 35 mins, **Servings**: 4
Yield: 4 servings

Ingredients

2 8-ounce of boneless, skinless chicken breasts

12 ounces of baby Yukon Gold potatoes, halved lengthwise

8 ounces of carrots, diagonally sliced into 1-inch pieces

3 tablespoons of extra-virgin olive oil, divided

2 teaspoons of ground coriander, divided

¾ teaspoon of salt, divided

½ teaspoon of ground pepper, divided

2 tablespoons of lemon juice

2 tablespoons of chopped shallot

1 tablespoon of whole-grain Dijon mustard

2 teaspoons of honey

1 pound of fresh asparagus, trimmed

2 tablespoons of chopped fresh flat-leaf parsley

1 tablespoon of chopped fresh dill

Lemon wedges

Directions

Heat up the oven to 375°F. Put the chicken on a clean surface and cover it with plastic wrap. Use a meat mallet to make the chicken pieces even and ½-inch thick. Put them on one side of a big baking sheet with edges.

Put the potatoes and carrots in one layer on the other side of the pan. Pour 1 tablespoon of oil over the chicken and vegetables; sprinkle 1 teaspoon of coriander, ½ teaspoon of salt and ¼ teaspoon of pepper. Bake for 15 minutes.

In a small bowl, whisk lemon juice, shallot, mustard, honey and the rest of the oil, coriander, salt and pepper.

Take out the pan from the oven; change the oven to broil. Mix the potato-carrot mixture; put asparagus in the middle of the pan.Spoon the lemon juice-shallot mixture over the chicken and vegetables.

Broil until the chicken and vegetables are a little brown, asparagus is crunchy-soft and a thermometer in the thickest part of the chicken shows 165°F, about 10 minutes. Take out from oven; sprinkle with parsley and dill. Eat with lemon slices.

Treat and Snack Recipes

- Peanut Butter-Banana Cinnamon Toast
- Homemade Trail Mix
- Air-Fryer Plantains
- Apricot-Ginger Energy Balls
- Air-Fryer Sweet Potato Chips
- Blueberry Almond Chia Pudding
- Apricot-Sunflower Granola Bars
- Zucchini Mini Muffins
- Rosemary-Garlic Pecans
- Avocado Hummus
- Avocado-Yogurt Dip

Peanut Butter-Banana Cinnamon Toast

Nutrition Facts ‖ Fat **9g**, Carb **38g**, Protein **8g**, Fiber **6g**, Calories **266**
Prep Time: 5 mins, **Total Time**: 5 mins, **Servings**: 1
Yield: 1 serving

Ingredients
1 slice of whole-wheat bread, toasted
1 tablespoon of peanut butter
1 small banana, sliced
Cinnamon, to taste

Directions
Put peanut butter on toast and add banana slices on top. Add some cinnamon as you like.

Homemade Trail Mix

Nutrition Facts || Fat **7g**, Carb **15g**, Protein **4g**, Fiber **3g**, Calories **132**
Cook Time: 5 mins, **Total Time**: 5 mins, **Servings**: 5
Yield: 5 servings

Ingredients
¼ cup of whole shelled (unpeeled) almonds
¼ cup of unsalted dry-roasted peanuts
¼ cup of dried cranberries
¼ cup of chopped pitted dates
2 ounces of dried apricots, or other dried fruit

Directions
Mix peanuts, almonds, dates, cranberries and apricots (or other fruit) in a medium bowl.

Tips
Keep them in plastic bags at room temperature for up to 2 weeks.

Air-Fryer Plantains

Nutrition Facts ‖ Fat **7g**, Carb **29g**, Protein **1g**, Fiber **2g**, Calories **171**
Active Time: 15 mins, **Total Time**: 55 mins, **Servings**: 4
Yield: 4 servings

Ingredients

2 medium ripe plantains (about 1 ¼ pounds total), peeled and sliced (1/2-inch)
2 tablespoons of avocado oil, divided
¼ teaspoon of salt

Directions

Heat up the air fryer to 360°F for 10 minutes. Spray the fryer basket with cooking spray a lot. Put plantains and 1 tablespoon of oil in a medium bowl and toss them. Put the plantains in one layer in the fryer basket. You may have to do it in parts. Cook for 5 minutes; turn the plantains over and keep cooking until they are crispy and brown, 6 to 8 minutes more. Move the plantains to a cutting board carefully.

Use the bottom of a small bowl or pan to press each plantain slice into a flat circle (about ¼-inch thick); move them to a medium bowl. Toss the flat plantains with the rest of the oil. Put the plantains back in the fryer basket in one layer. You may have to do it in parts again. Cook until they have some crisp spots, 5 to 7 minutes. Add some salt and eat right away.

Apricot-Ginger Energy Balls

Nutrition Facts || Fat **3g**, Carb **8g**, Protein **1g**, Fiber **1g**, Calories **57**
Prep Time: 25 mins, **Total Time**: 25 mins, **Servings**: 32
Yield: 32 balls

Ingredients

1 ½ cups of dried apricots
¾ cup of rolled oats
¾ cup of finely shredded unsweetened coconut
6 tablespoons of tahini
3 tablespoons of honey
¾ teaspoon of ground ginger
A pinch of salt

Directions

Put apricots, oats, coconut, tahini, honey, ginger and salt in a food processor. Pulse until they are chopped well, 10 to 20 times, then blend for about 1 minute, scraping the sides if needed, until the mix is crumbly but can stick together to make a ball.

Use wet hands (so the mix doesn't stick to them), squeeze about 1 tablespoon of the mix hard between your hands and roll into a ball. Put it in a container. Do the same with the rest of the mix.

Tips

Keep them in the fridge for up to 1 week or freeze them for up to 3 months.

Air-Fryer Sweet Potato Chips

Nutrition Facts || Fat **2g**, Carb **4g**, Protein **0g**, Fiber **1g**, Calories **31**
Prep Time: 5 mins, **Additional Time**: 55 mins
Total Time: 1 hr, **Servings**: 8
Yield: 8 servings

Ingredients

1 medium sweet potato, (about 8 ounces), sliced into 1/8-inch-thick rounds
1 tablespoon of canola oil
¼ teaspoon of sea salt
¼ teaspoon of ground pepper

Directions

Put sweet potato slices in a big bowl of cold water; let them soak for 20 minutes. Take them out and dry them with paper towels.

Put the sweet potatoes back in the dry bowl. Add oil, salt and pepper; gently stir to coat.

Spray the air-fryer basket with cooking spray a little. Put some of the sweet potatoes in the basket in one layer. Cook at 350 degrees F until they are done and crispy, about 15 minutes, turning and moving them into one layer every 5 minutes. Use tongs to carefully take the chips out of the air fryer to a plate. Do the same with the rest of the sweet potatoes.

Cool the chips for 5 minutes; eat right away or cool them completely and keep them in a closed plastic container for up to 3 days.

Blueberry Almond Chia Pudding

Nutrition Facts || Fat **11g**, Carb **30g**, Protein **6g**, Fiber **10g**, Calories **229**
Prep Time: 10 mins, **Additional Time**: 8 hrs
Total Time: 8 hrs 10 mins, **Servings**: 1
Yield: 1 cup

Ingredients

½ cup of unsweetened almond milk or other non dairy milk beverage

2 tablespoons of chia seeds

2 teaspoons of pure maple syrup

⅛ teaspoon of almond extract

½ cup of fresh blueberries, divided

1 tablespoon of toasted slivered almonds, divided

Directions

Mix almond milk (or other non-dairy milk drink), chia, maple syrup and almond extract in a small bowl. Cover and keep it in the fridge for at least 8 hours and up to 3 days.

When you want to eat it, stir the pudding well. Put about half the pudding in a glass (or bowl) and add half the blueberries and almonds. Put the rest of the pudding and add the rest of the blueberries and almonds.

Tips

Keep the pudding (Step 1) in the fridge for up to 3 days. Do Step 2 just before eating.

Apricot-Sunflower Granola Bars

Nutrition Facts ‖ Fat **6g**, Carb **22g**, Protein **4g**, Fiber **2g**, Calories **152**
Prep Time: 20 mins, **Additional Time**: 1hr 10 mins
Total Time: 1 hr 30 mins, **Servings**: 1
Yield: 24 bars

Ingredients

3 cups of old-fashioned rolled oats

1 cup of crispy brown rice cereal

1 cup of finely chopped dried apricots (1/4 inch)

½ cup of unsalted pepitas, toasted

½ cup of unsalted sunflower seeds, toasted

¼ teaspoon of salt

⅔ cup of brown rice syrup or light corn syrup

½ cup of sunflower seed butter

1 teaspoon of ground cinnamon

Directions

Heat up the oven to 325 degrees F. Put parchment paper on a 9-by-13-inch baking pan with extra parchment hanging over two sides. Spray the parchment with cooking spray a little.

Mix oats, rice cereal, apricots, pepitas, sunflower seeds and salt in a big bowl.

Put rice syrup (or corn syrup), sunflower butter and cinnamon in a bowl that can go in the microwave. Microwave it for 30 seconds (or heat it in a pot over medium heat for 1 minute). Add it to the dry mix and stir until they are mixed well. Move it to the pan and press it into the pan with the back of a spatula.

For softer bars, bake until the edge starts to get some color and the middle is still soft, 20 to 25 minutes. For harder bars, bake until the edge is golden brown and the middle is kind of hard, 30 to 35 minutes. (Both will still be soft when warm and get harder as they cool.)

Let it cool in the pan for 10 minutes, then use the parchment to help you, take it out of the pan onto a cutting board (it will still be soft). Cut it into 24 bars, then let it cool completely without moving the bars, about 30 minutes more. When they are cool, separate them into bars.

Tips
Wrap them tight and keep them for up to 1 week at room temperature.

Zucchini Mini Muffins

Nutrition Facts ‖ Fat **8g**, Carb **30g**, Protein **3g**, Fiber **2g**, Calories **196**
Prep Time: 15 mins, **Additional Time**: 45 mins
Total Time: 1 hr, **Servings**: 12
Yield: 24 mini muffins

Ingredients

¾ cup of all-purpose flour
¾ cup of white whole-wheat flour
1 teaspoon of ground cinnamon
¾ teaspoon of baking soda
½ teaspoon of salt
2 large eggs
¾ cup of sugar
¼ cup of canola oil or unsalted butter, melted
1 ½ teaspoons of vanilla extract
2 cups of shredded and coarsely chopped zucchini
½ cup of mini chocolate chips

Directions

Heat up the oven to 350 degrees F. Spray a 24-cup mini muffin tin with cooking spray.

In a big bowl, whisk both flours, cinnamon, baking soda and salt. In a medium bowl, whisk eggs, sugar, oil (or butter) and vanilla. Add zucchini and chocolate chips and stir. Add the wet mix to the flour mix and stir until they are mixed well. Put the batter in the muffin tin. Bake until a toothpick in the middle of a muffin comes out clean, about 10 minutes. Let it cool in the tin for 5 minutes, then take it out and put it on a rack to cool completely.

Tips

You can keep them in a tight container at room temperature for up to 2 days or wrap them in plastic and freeze them for up to 1 month.

Rosemary-Garlic Pecans

Nutrition Facts || Fat **18g**, Carb **4g**, Protein **3g**, Fiber **3g**, Calories **175**
Active Time: 5 mins, **Total Time**: 1hr 20 mins, **Servings**: 12
Yield: 12 ¼-cups

Ingredients
1 large egg white
3 tablespoons of dried rosemary, finely chopped
2 teaspoons of garlic salt
3 cups of pecans

Directions
Preheat oven to 250°F.

In a medium bowl, whisk egg white, rosemary and garlic salt. Put pecans in and toss them to coat. Put them in one layer on a big baking sheet with edges.

Bake them, stirring every 15 minutes, until they are dry, about 45 minutes. Let them cool completely before keeping them, about 30 minutes.

Tips
You can keep them in a tight container for up to 2 weeks.

Avocado Hummus

Nutrition Facts ‖ Fat **12g**, Carb **10g**, Protein **3g**, Fiber **3g**, Calories **156**
Prep Time: 10 mins, **Total Time**: 10 mins, **Servings**: 10
Yield: 10

Ingredients

1 (15 ounce) can of no-salt-added chickpeas
1 ripe avocado, halved and pitted
1 cup of fresh cilantro leaves
¼ cup of tahini
¼ cup of extra-virgin olive oil
¼ cup of lemon juice
1 clove of garlic
1 teaspoon of ground cumin
½ teaspoon of salt

Directions

Pour out the chickpeas, keeping 2 tablespoons of the liquid. Put the chickpeas and the liquid in a food processor. Add avocado, cilantro, tahini, oil, lemon juice, garlic, cumin and salt. Blend until it's very smooth. Eat with veggie chips, pita chips or crudités.

Avocado-Yogurt Dip

Nutrition Facts ‖ Fat **4g**, Carb **4g**, Protein **1g**, Fiber **2g**, Calories **51**
Cook Time: 10 mins, **Total Time**: 10 mins, **Servings**: 8
Yield: 8 servings

Ingredients

1 ripe avocado, peeled and pitted
½ cup of nonfat plain yogurt
⅓ cup of packed fresh cilantro leaves
2 tablespoons of chopped onion
1 tablespoon of lime juice
¼ teaspoon of salt
¼ teaspoon of freshly ground pepper
Hot sauce to taste, optional

Directions

Put avocado, yogurt, cilantro, onion, lime juice, salt and pepper in a food processor. Blend until it's smooth. Add hot sauce, if you like.

Tips

You can keep it covered in the fridge for up to 2 days.

Salad Recipes

- Mason Jar Power Salad with Chickpeas & Tuna
- Breakfast Salad with Egg & Salsa Verde Vinaigrette
- Quinoa, Avocado & Chickpea Salad over Mixed Greens
- No-Cook Black Bean Salad
- Spinach & Strawberry Meal-Prep Salad
- Superfood Chopped Salad with Salmon & Creamy Garlic Dressing
- Chicken & Shredded Brussels Sprout Salad with Bacon Vinaigrette
- Salmon Couscous Salad
- Chicken with Spinach & Tomato Orzo Salad
- Quinoa Power Salad

Mason Jar Power Salad with Chickpeas & Tuna

Nutrition Facts || Fat **23g**, Carb **30g**, Protein **26g**, Fiber **9g**, Calories **430**
Prep Time: 5 mins, **Total Time**: 5 mins, **Servings**: 1
Yield: 4 cups

Ingredients
3 cups of bite-sized pieces chopped kale
2 tablespoons of honey-mustard vinaigrette
1 2.5-ounce of pouch tuna in water
½ cup of rinsed canned chickpeas
1 carrot, peeled and shredded

Directions
Mix kale and dressing in a bowl, then put them in a 1-quart mason jar. Add tuna, chickpeas and carrot on top. Close the lid and keep the jar in the fridge for up to 2 days.

To eat, pour the jar into a bowl and mix the salad ingredients with the kale with dressing.

Tips
Store in the fridge for up to 2 days.

Breakfast Salad with Egg & Salsa Verde Vinaigrette

Nutrition Facts || Fat **34g**, Carb **37g**, Protein **16g**, Fiber **13g**, Calories **527**
Prep Time: 10 mins, **Total Time**: 10 mins, **Servings**: 1
Yield: 1 serving

Ingredients

3 tablespoons of salsa verde, such as Frontera brand
1 tablespoon plus 1 tsp. of extra-virgin olive oil, divided
2 tablespoons of chopped cilantro, plus more for garnish
2 cups of mesclun or other salad greens
8 blue corn tortilla chips, broken into large pieces
½ cup of canned red kidney beans, rinsed
¼ avocado, sliced
1 large egg

Directions

In a small bowl, whisk salsa, 1 Tbsp. of oil, and cilantro. Mix half of it with mesclun (or other greens) in a big bowl for serving.

Put chips, beans, and avocado on the salad.

Heat the rest of the oil in a small nonstick pan over medium-high heat. Fry the egg until the white is done but the yolk is still a bit runny, about 2 minutes.

Put the egg on the salad. Pour the rest of the salsa vinaigrette over it and add more cilantro, if you like.

Quinoa, Avocado & Chickpea Salad over Mixed Greens

Nutrition Facts || Fat **32g**, Carb **47g**, Protein **12g**, Fiber **13g**, Calories **501**
Prep Time: 20 mins, **Total Time**: 25 mins, **Servings**: 2
Yield: 5 cups

Ingredients

⅔ cup of water

⅓ cup of quinoa

¼ teaspoon of kosher salt or other coarse salt

1 clove of garlic, crushed and peeled

2 teaspoons of grated lemon zest

3 tablespoons of lemon juice

3 tablespoons of olive oil

¼ teaspoon of ground pepper

1 cup of rinsed no-salt-added canned chickpeas

1 medium carrot, shredded (1/2 cup)

½ avocado, diced

1 (5 ounce) of package prewashed mixed greens, such as spring mix or baby kale-spinach blend (8 cups packed)

Directions

Boil water in a small pot. Add quinoa. Turn down the heat to low, cover, and let it simmer until it absorbs all the water, about 15 minutes. Use a fork to make the grains fluffy and separate; let it cool for 5 minutes.

While that's happening, sprinkle salt on garlic on a cutting board. Use the side of a spoon to mash the garlic until it becomes a paste. Put it in a medium bowl. Whisk in lemon zest, lemon juice, oil, and pepper. Take 3 Tbsp. of the dressing and put it in a small bowl and keep it aside.

Put chickpeas, carrot, and avocado in the bowl with the rest of the dressing; gently mix them together. Let it sit for 5 minutes to let the flavors mix. Add the quinoa and gently stir to coat.

Put greens in a big bowl and toss them with the 3 Tbsp. dressing you kept aside. Split the greens between 2 plates and put the quinoa mixture on top.

Tips
Make quinoa (Step 1) and keep it in the fridge for up to 2 days.

No-Cook Black Bean Salad

Nutrition Facts ‖ Fat **16g**, Carb **41g**, Protein **11g**, Fiber **13g**, Calories **322**
Prep Time: 30 mins, **Total Time**: 30 mins, **Servings**: 4
Yield: 8 cups

Ingredients

½ cup of thinly sliced red onion

1 medium ripe avocado, pitted and roughly chopped

¼ cup of cilantro leaves

¼ cup of lime juice

2 tablespoons of extra-virgin olive oil

1 clove of garlic, minced

½ teaspoon of salt

8 cups of mixed salad greens

2 medium ears of corn, kernels removed, or 2 cups frozen corn, thawed and patted dry

1 pint of grape tomatoes, halved

1 (15 ounce) can of black beans, rinsed

Directions

Put onion in a medium bowl and fill it with cold water. Leave it there. Put avocado, cilantro, lime juice, oil, garlic and salt in a small food processor. Blend, scraping the sides if needed, until it's smooth and creamy.

Right before eating, put salad greens, corn, tomatoes and beans in a big bowl. Pour out the water from the onions and add them to the bowl, alongside the avocado dressing. Mix well.

Spinach & Strawberry Meal-Prep Salad

Nutrition Facts || Fat **24g**, Carb **14g**, Protein **26g**, Fiber **5g**, Calories **374**
Prep Time: 15 mins, **Total Time**: 30 mins, **Servings**: 4
Yield: 4 servings

Ingredients

1 pound of boneless, skinless chicken thighs
½ teaspoon of kosher salt
½ teaspoon of dried thyme
½ teaspoon of ground pepper
8 cups of baby spinach
2 cups of sliced strawberries
¼ cup of feta cheese (Optional)
¼ cup of chopped toasted walnuts
6 tablespoons of Balsamic Vinaigrette

Directions

Heat up the oven to 400 degrees F. Put parchment or foil on a baking sheet. Put the chicken on the baking sheet. Sprinkle salt, thyme and pepper all over it. Roast it, turning it once, until the chicken is done and has a temperature of 165°F, 15 to 17 minutes. Let it cool down, then cut it into small pieces.

Split spinach into 4 containers with lids (2 cups each). Put one-fourth of the chicken pieces, ½ cup of sliced strawberries, 1 tablespoon of feta (if using) and 1 tablespoon of walnuts on each container. Close the salad containers and keep them in the fridge for up to 4 days. Put 1 ½ tablespoons of vinaigrette in each of 4 small containers with lids and keep them in the fridge for up to 5 days. Add the vinaigrette to the salads just before eating.

Tips
Keep the salad in the fridge for up to 4 days, but don't slice and add strawberries (and feta if using) until you are ready to eat.

Superfood Chopped Salad with Salmon & Creamy Garlic Dressing

Nutrition Facts || Fat **24g**, Carb **19g**, Protein **32g**, Fiber **6g**, Calories **409**
Prep Time: 30 mins, **Total Time**: 30 mins, **Servings**: 4
Yield: 4 servings

Ingredients

1 pound of salmon fillet
½ cup of low-fat plain yogurt
¼ cup of mayonnaise
2 tablespoons of lemon juice
2 tablespoons of grated Parmesan cheese
1 tablespoon of finely chopped fresh parsley
1 tablespoon of snipped fresh chives
2 teaspoons of reduced-sodium tamari or soy sauce
1 medium clove of garlic, minced
¼ teaspoon of ground pepper
8 cups of chopped curly kale
2 cups of chopped broccoli
2 cups of chopped red cabbage
2 cups of finely diced carrots
½ cup of sunflower seeds, toasted

Directions

Put the rack in the top part of the oven. Turn on the broiler to high. Put foil on a baking sheet. Put the salmon on the baking sheet, skin-side down. Broil it, turning the pan around once, until the salmon is cooked in the middle, 8 to 12 minutes. Cut it into 4 pieces.

While that's happening, whisk yogurt, mayonnaise, lemon juice, Parmesan, parsley, chives, tamari (or soy sauce), garlic and pepper in a small bowl. Mix kale, broccoli, cabbage, carrots and sunflower seeds in a big bowl. Add ¾ cup of the dressing and mix to coat. Split the salad into 4 plates and put a piece of salmon and about 1 tablespoon of the rest of the dressing on each plate.

Chicken & Shredded Brussels Sprout Salad with Bacon Vinaigrette

Nutrition Facts || Fat **12g**, Carb **28g**, Protein **34g**, Fiber **7g**, Calories **357**
Prep Time: 40 mins, **Total Time**: 40 mins, **Servings**: 4
Yield: 8 cups

Ingredients

4 slices of center-cut bacon (1 ounce)
2 tablespoons of extra-virgin olive oil
1 large shallot, minced (1/4 cup)
2 tablespoons of red-wine vinegar
1 teaspoon of honey
½ teaspoon of Dijon mustard
½ teaspoon of salt
½ teaspoon of ground pepper
1 pound of Brussels sprouts, trimmed and shredded (6 cups)
2 medium Fuji apples, thinly sliced
2 cups of shredded cooked chicken breast (12 ounces)

Directions

Fry bacon in a big nonstick pan over medium heat until it's crispy, 5 to 7 minutes. Move it to a plate with paper towels to soak up the grease. Break it into big pieces and keep it aside.

Leave 1 tablespoon of bacon grease in the pan. Add oil and heat it over medium heat. Add shallot and cook it, stirring, until it's soft and light brown, 1 to 2 minutes. Turn off the heat.

Put vinegar, honey, mustard, salt, and pepper in the pan and whisk them together. Put Brussels sprouts in and toss them to coat. Keep tossing them sometimes until they get a little soft from the heat left in the pan, 2 to 3 minutes.

Mix apples and chicken in a big bowl. Add the Brussels sprouts and any dressing left in the pan and gently stir them together. Split them into 4 bowls and eat them with the bacon on top.

Tips

To make Brussels sprouts into shreds, first use a knife to cut off any hard stems. Then use the knife or the food processor with a slicing blade to cut the sprouts (see below). To make it easier, buy sliced Brussels sprouts from the store.

• To use a chef's knife: Cut Brussels sprouts in half from top to bottom. Put the cut-side down on a cutting board and slice them thinly. Pull apart the slices into shreds.

• To use a food processor: Put a slicing blade in a food processor and, while it's running, drop the sprouts in the food chute. Pull apart the slices into shreds, if needed.

Salmon Couscous Salad

Nutrition Facts ‖ Fat **22g**, Carb **35g**, Protein **35g**, Fiber **6g**, Calories **464**
Prep Time: 10 mins, **Total Time**: 10 mins, **Servings**: 1
Yield: 4 cups

Ingredients

¼ cup of sliced cremini mushrooms
¼ cup of diced eggplant
3 cups of baby spinach
2 tablespoons of white-wine vinaigrette, divided
¼ cup of cooked Israeli couscous, preferably whole-wheat
4 ounces of cooked salmon
¼ cup of sliced dried apricots
2 tablespoons of crumbled goat cheese (1/2 ounce)

Directions

Spray a small pan with cooking spray and heat it over medium-high heat. Put mushrooms and eggplant in and cook them, stirring, until they are lightly browned and have some juice, 3 to 5 minutes. Take it off the heat and keep it aside.

Mix spinach with 1 Tbsp. plus 1 tsp. of vinaigrette and put it on a 9-inch plate.

Mix couscous with the rest of the vinaigrette and put it on the spinach. Put salmon on it. Put the cooked vegetables, dried apricots, and goat cheese on top.

Tips

Whisk 2 Tbsp. of white-wine vinegar with 1/8 tsp. each of salt and pepper, to make a quick white-wine vinaigrette. Slowly whisk in ¼ cup of extra-virgin olive oil until it's mixed. You can keep the extra dressing, covered, in the fridge for up to 5 days. Before using, bring it to room temperature.

Chicken with Spinach & Tomato Orzo Salad

Nutrition Facts ‖ Fat **8g**, Carb **28g**, Protein **32g**, Fiber **6g**, Calories **402**
Prep Time: 40 mins, **Total Time**: 40 mins, **Servings**: 4
Yield: 4 servings

Ingredients

2 skinless, boneless chicken breasts (8 ounces each), halved
3 tablespoons of extra-virgin olive oil, divided
1 teaspoon of lemon zest
½ teaspoon of salt, divided
½ teaspoon of ground pepper, divided
¾ cup of whole-wheat orzo
2 cups of thinly sliced baby spinach
1 cup of chopped cucumber
1 cup of chopped tomato
¼ cup of chopped red onion
¼ cup of crumbled feta cheese
2 tablespoons of chopped Kalamata olives
2 tablespoons of lemon juice
1 clove of garlic, grated
2 teaspoons of chopped fresh oregano

Directions

Heat up the oven to 425 degrees F.

Rub chicken with 1 tablespoon of oil and sprinkle with lemon zest and ¼ teaspoon each of salt and pepper. Put it in a baking dish. Bake it until a thermometer in the thickest part shows 165 degrees F, 25 to 30 minutes.

While that's happening, boil a quart of water in a medium pot over high heat. Put orzo in and cook for 8 minutes. Put spinach in and cook for 1 more minute. Drain and rinse with cold water. Drain well and move to a big bowl. Add cucumber, tomato, onion, feta and olives. Stir them together.

In a small bowl, whisk the rest of the oil, lemon juice, garlic, oregano and the rest of the salt and pepper. Stir all but 1 tablespoon of the dressing into the orzo mix. Pour the rest of the dressing over the chicken and eat it with the salad.

Quinoa Power Salad

Nutrition Facts || Fat **21g**, Carb **35g**, Protein **29g**, Fiber **6g**, Calories **466**
Prep Time: 20 mins, **Additional Time**: 20 mins
Total Time: 40mins, **Servings**: 2
Yield: 2 servings

Ingredients

1 medium sweet potato, peeled and cut into ½-inch-thick wedges

½ red onion, cut into ¼-inch-thick wedges

2 tablespoons of extra-virgin olive oil, divided

½ teaspoon of garlic powder

¼ teaspoon of salt, divided

8 ounces of chicken tenders

2 tablespoons of whole-grain mustard, divided

1 tablespoon of finely chopped shallot

1 tablespoon of pure maple syrup

1 tablespoon of cider vinegar

4 cups of baby greens, such as spinach, kale and/or arugula, washed and dried

½ cup of cooked red quinoa, cooled

1 tablespoon of unsalted sunflower seeds, toasted

Directions

Heat the oven to 425°F. In a medium bowl, mix sweet potato and onion with 1 tablespoon of oil, garlic powder and a pinch of salt. Arrange them on a large baking sheet with edges and bake for 15 minutes.

In the meantime, put chicken and 1 tablespoon of mustard in the same bowl and stir well. After the vegetables have baked for 15 minutes, take them out of the oven and give them a stir. Put the chicken on the same pan and bake for another 10 minutes or until the vegetables start to brown and the chicken is done. Take them out of the oven and let them cool down.

While the chicken is cooling, combine shallot, maple syrup, vinegar and the remaining 1 tablespoon of oil, 1 tablespoon of mustard and a pinch of salt in the large bowl and whisk well.

Shred the chicken when it is cool enough and add it to the bowl with the dressing. Also add baby greens, quinoa and the roasted vegetables. Mix everything with the dressing and sprinkle with sunflower seeds.

Tips
Prepare up to Step 3 two days in advance. Keep the vegetables, chicken and dressing in separate containers in the fridge. Mix them just before serving.

Smoothie Recipes

- Berry-Almond Smoothie Bowl
- Pineapple Green Smoothie
- Chocolate-Banana Protein Smoothie
- Perfect Green Smoothie
- Fruit & Yogurt Smoothie
- Mango-Ginger Smoothie
- Cantaloupe Smoothie
- Strawberry-Blueberry-Banana Smoothie
- Strawberry-Chocolate Smoothie
- Banana-Cocoa Soy Smoothie

Berry-Almond Smoothie Bowl

Nutrition Facts || Fat **19g**, Carb **36g**, Protein **9g**, Fiber **14g**, Calories **360**
Prep Time: 10 mins, **Total Time**: 10 mins, **Servings**: 1
Yield: 1 serving

Ingredients
⅔ cup of frozen raspberries
½ cup of frozen sliced banana
½ cup of plain unsweetened almond milk
5 tablespoons of sliced almonds, divided
¼ teaspoon of ground cinnamon
⅛ teaspoon of ground cardamom
⅛ teaspoon of vanilla extract
¼ cup of blueberries
1 tablespoon of unsweetened coconut flakes

Directions
Put raspberries, banana, almond milk, 3 tablespoons of almonds, cinnamon, cardamom and vanilla in a blender and blend until very smooth.

Transfer the smoothie to a bowl and add blueberries, coconut and the remaining 2 tablespoons of almonds on top.

Pineapple Green Smoothie

Nutrition Facts || Fat **6g**, Carb **54g**, Protein **13g**, Fiber **10g**, Calories **297**
Active Time: 5 mins, **Total Time**: 5 mins, **Servings**: 1
Yield: 1 serving

Ingredients

½ cup of unsweetened almond milk
⅓ cup of nonfat plain Greek yogurt
1 cup of baby spinach
1 cup of frozen banana slices (about 1 medium banana)
½ cup of frozen pineapple chunks
1 tablespoon of chia seeds
1-2 teaspoons of pure maple syrup or honey (optional)

Directions

Put almond milk and yogurt in a blender first, then add spinach, banana, pineapple, chia seeds and sweetener (if using) and blend until smooth.

Chocolate-Banana Protein Smoothie

Nutrition Facts ‖ Fat **2g**, Carb **64g**, Protein **15g**, Fiber **9g**, Calories **310**
Prep Time: 5 mins, **Total Time**: 5 mins, **Servings**: 1
Yield: 1 serving

Ingredients
1 banana, frozen
½ cup of cooked red lentils
½ cup of nonfat milk
2 teaspoons of unsweetened cocoa powder
1 teaspoon of pure maple syrup

Directions
Put banana, lentils, milk, cocoa and syrup in a blender and blend until smooth.

Perfect Green Smoothie

Nutrition Facts ‖ Fat **14g**, Carb **55g**, Protein **6g**, Fiber **12g**, Calories **343**
Prep Time: 5 mins, **Total Time**: 5 mins, **Servings**: 1
Yield: 1 serving

Ingredients

1 large ripe banana
1 cup of packed baby kale or coarsely chopped mature kale
1 cup of unsweetened vanilla almond milk
¼ ripe avocado
1 tablespoon of chia seeds
2 teaspoons of honey
1 cup of ice cubes

Directions

In a blender, add banana, kale, almond milk, avocado, chia seeds and honey. Blend until creamy and smooth. Add ice and blend some more until smooth.

Fruit & Yogurt Smoothie

Nutrition Facts || Fat **2g**, Carb **56g**, Protein **12g**, Fiber **7g**, Calories **279**
Active Time: 10 mins, **Total Time**: 10 mins, **Servings**: 1
Yield: 1 serving

Ingredients

¾ cup of nonfat plain yogurt
½ cup of 100% pure fruit juice
1 ½ cups (6 ½ ounces) of frozen fruit, such as blueberries, raspberries, pineapple or peaches

Directions

Blend yogurt and juice until smooth in a blender. While the blender is still running, add the fruit through the lid opening and keep blending until smooth.

Mango-Ginger Smoothie

Nutrition Facts || Fat **1g**, Carb **79g**, Protein **12g**, Fiber **10g**, Calories **352**
Cook Time: 10 mins, **Total Time**: 10 mins, **Servings**: 1
Yield: 1 serving

Ingredients

½ cup of cooked red lentils, cooled
1 cup of frozen mango chunks
¾ cup of carrot juice
1 teaspoon of chopped fresh ginger
1 teaspoon of honey
A pinch of ground cardamom, plus more for garnish
3 ice cubes

Directions

Put lentils, mango, carrot juice, ginger, honey, cardamom and ice cubes in a blender and blend until very smooth, for about 2 to 3 minutes. Sprinkle more cardamom on top if you like.

Tips

To make red lentils: Boil them until they are just soft, about 15 minutes. Drain and let them cool. (1 cup dry = 2 ½ cups cooked.) Keep them in the fridge for up to 3 days. Or freeze them in ½-cup portions for up to 3 months (defrost before using).

Cantaloupe Smoothie

Nutrition Facts || Fat **3g**, Carb **75g**, Protein **14g**, Fiber **6g**, Calories **364**
Cook Time: 10 mins, **Total Time**: 10 mins, **Servings**: 1
Yield: 1 serving

Ingredients

1 banana
2 cups of chopped ripe cantaloupe
½ cup of nonfat or low-fat plain yogurt
2 tablespoons of nonfat dry milk
1 ½ tablespoons of frozen orange juice concentrate
½ teaspoon of vanilla extract

Directions

Put the banana in the freezer with the peel on overnight (or for up to 3 months).

Take the banana out of the freezer and wait until the skin starts to soften, about 2 minutes. Peel the banana with a small knife. (It's OK if some fiber stays on.) Cut the banana into pieces. Put them in a blender or food processor with cantaloupe, yogurt, dry milk, orange juice and vanilla. Blend until smooth.

Strawberry-Blueberry-Banana Smoothie

Nutrition Facts || Fat **17g**, Carb **46g**, Protein **7g**, Fiber **7g**, Calories **335**
Prep Time: 5 mins, **Total Time**: 5 mins, **Servings**: 1
Yield: 2 cups

Ingredients
½ cup of frozen strawberries
½ cup of frozen blueberries
1 small ripe banana (frozen, if desired)
¾ cup of chilled unsweetened cashew milk, plus more if needed
1 tablespoon of cashew butter
1 tablespoon of hulled hemp seeds

Directions
Put strawberries, blueberries, banana, cashew milk, cashew butter and hemp seeds in a blender and blend until smooth. You may need to add more cashew milk to get the consistency you want. Enjoy right away.

Strawberry-Chocolate Smoothie

Nutrition Facts || Fat **13g**, Carb **47g**, Protein **7g**, Fiber **9g**, Calories **303**
Prep Time: 5 mins, **Total Time**: 5 mins, **Servings**: 1
Yield: 2 cups

Ingredients

1 ½ cups of frozen strawberries
1 cup of chilled unsweetened chocolate almond milk, plus more if needed
1 tablespoon of almond butter
1 tablespoon of unsweetened cocoa powder
1 tablespoon of honey

Directions

In a blender, add strawberries, almond milk, almond butter, cocoa and honey and blend until smooth. You may need to add more almond milk to get the consistency you want. Enjoy right away.

Banana-Cocoa Soy Smoothie

Nutrition Facts || Fat **8g**, Carb **62g**, Protein **16g**, Fiber **10g**, Calories **342**
Cook Time: 5 mins, **Additional Time**: 55 mins
Total Time: 1 hr, **Servings**: 1
Yield: 1 serving

Ingredients

1 banana
½ cup of silken tofu
½ cup of soymilk
2 tablespoons of unsweetened cocoa powder
1 tablespoon of honey

Directions

Cut the banana into pieces and freeze them until they are hard. In a blender, mix tofu, soymilk, cocoa and honey until smooth. While the blender is still running, add the frozen banana pieces through the lid opening and keep blending until smooth.

Weight loss Recipes

- Fresh Fruit Salad
- White Bean & Avocado Toast
- Strawberry & Yogurt Parfait
- Air-Fryer Crispy Chickpeas
- Rice Cake Snackwich
- Sprouted-Grain Toast with Peanut Butter & Banana
- Tasty Guacamole
- Kale Chips
- Bagel Gone Bananas
- Crunchy Roasted Chickpeas
- Banana & Walnut

Fresh Fruit Salad

Nutrition Facts || Fat **0g**, Carb **14g**, Protein **1g**, Fiber **3g**, Calories **57**
Active Time: 30 mins, **Total Time**: 30 mins, **Servings**: 10
Yield: 10 servings

Ingredients

Fruit Salad:
2 cups of diced fresh pineapple
1 pound of strawberries, hulled and sliced
½ pint of blackberries, halved
4 ripe kiwis, peeled, halved and sliced

Lime Yogurt Dressing (optional):
1 cup of low-fat plain yogurt
1 tablespoon of granulated sugar
2 teaspoons of lime zest
2 teaspoons of lime juice

Directions

For the dressing, if using: Mix yogurt, sugar, lime zest and lime juice in a medium bowl.

For the salad: Put pineapple, strawberries, blackberries and kiwi in a large bowl. Enjoy with lime yogurt dressing, if you like.

Tips

keep the fruit salad in the fridge for up to 2 hours. keep the dressing in the fridge for up to 1 day.

White Bean & Avocado Toast

Nutrition Facts || Fat **9g**, Carb **35g**, Protein **12g**, Fiber **11g**, Calories **230**
Prep Time: 5 mins, **Total Time**: 5 mins, **Servings**: 1
Yield: 1 slice

Ingredients

1 slice of whole-wheat bread, toasted

¼ avocado, mashed

½ cup of canned white beans, rinsed and drained

Kosher salt to taste

Ground pepper to taste

1 pinch of crushed red pepper

Directions

Spread avocado and white beans over toast. Add a pinch of salt, pepper and red pepper flakes for seasoning.

Strawberry & Yogurt Parfait

Nutrition Facts ‖ Fat **8g**, Carb **37g**, Protein **17g**, Fiber **6g**, Calories **285**
Active Time: 10 mins, **Total Time**: 10 mins, **Servings**: 1
Yield: 1 serving

Ingredients

1 cup of sliced fresh strawberries
1 teaspoon of sugar
½ cup of nonfat plain Greek yogurt
¼ cup of granola

Directions

Mix strawberries and sugar in a small bowl and wait until the juice comes out of the berries, about 5 minutes.

To make the parfait, put yogurt and the strawberries with their juice in a container that can hold 2 cups. Sprinkle granola on top.

Air-Fryer Crispy Chickpeas

Nutrition Facts ‖ Fat **6g**, Carb **14g**, Protein **5g**, Fiber **3g**, Calories **132**
Prep Time: 20 mins, **Total Time**: 20 mins, **Servings**: 4
Yield: 1 cup

Ingredients

1 (15 ounce) can of unsalted chickpeas, rinsed and drained
1 ½ tablespoons of toasted sesame oil
¼ teaspoon of smoked paprika
¼ teaspoon of crushed red pepper
⅛ teaspoon of salt
Cooking spray
2 lime wedges

Directions

Put chickpeas on some paper towels and cover with more paper towels. Press until they are very dry, rolling the chickpeas under the paper towels to dry all sides.

In a medium bowl, toss the chickpeas and oil together. Add paprika, red pepper flakes and salt. Put them in an air fryer basket and spray with cooking spray. Cook at 400 degrees F until they are very brown, 12 to 14 minutes, shaking the basket sometimes. Squeeze lime slices over the chickpeas and enjoy.

Rice Cake Snackwich

Nutrition Facts || Fat **10g**, Carb **31g**, Protein **5g**, Fiber **5g**, Calories **225**
Prep Time: 5 mins, **Total Time**: 5 mins, **Servings**: 1
Yield: 1 sandwich

Ingredients

1 tablespoon of almond butter
2 brown rice cakes
½ teaspoon of flaxseed
A pinch of ground cinnamon
½ apple, sliced

Directions

Put almond butter on one rice cake. Add flaxseed and cinnamon on top. Cover with apple and another rice cake.

Sprouted-Grain Toast with Peanut Butter & Banana

Nutrition Facts || Fat **9g**, Carb **45g**, Protein **9g**, Fiber **7g**, Calories **290**
Prep Time: 5 mins, **Total Time**: 5 mins, **Servings**: 1
Yield: 1 serving

Ingredients
1 slice of sprouted-grain bread
1 tablespoon of peanut butter
1 medium banana, sliced

Directions
Make the bread toast. Put peanut butter on the toast and add banana slices on top.

Tasty Guacamole

Nutrition Facts || Fat **11g**, Carb **85g**, Protein **2g**, Fiber **5g**, Calories **125**
Prep Time: 15 mins, **Total Time**: 15 mins, **Servings**: 8
Yield: 2 cups

Ingredients
3 medium ripe avocados
1 medium jalapeño pepper, finely chopped
¼ cup of finely chopped red or white onion
¼ cup of chopped fresh cilantro
2 tablespoons of lime juice
1 clove of garlic, grated
½ teaspoon of salt

Directions
In a medium bowl, use a fork to smash avocados. Mix in jalapeño, onion, cilantro, lime juice, garlic and salt until well combined.

Kale Chips

Nutrition Facts || Fat **5g**, Carb **16g**, Protein **5g**, Fiber **6g**, Calories **110**
Active Time: 25 mins, **Total Time**: 25 mins, **Servings**: 4
Yield: 4 servings

Ingredients

1 large bunch of kale, tough stems removed, leaves torn into pieces (about 16 cups)
1 tablespoon of extra-virgin olive oil
¼ teaspoon of salt

Directions

Put the racks in the top and middle of the oven and heat it to 400°F.

Make sure the kale is dry by patting it well with a clean kitchen towel; put it in a large bowl. Pour oil over the kale and sprinkle salt. Use your hands to rub the oil and salt on the kale leaves so they are coated evenly. Spread the kale on 2 large baking sheets with edges in one layer, without overlapping the leaves. (If you have too much kale, you can bake the chips in batches.)

Bake until most of the leaves are crispy, switching the pans from front to back and top to bottom halfway through, 8 to 12 minutes in total. (If you are baking only 1 sheet at a time, check after 8 minutes to avoid burning.)

Bagel Gone Bananas

Nutrition Facts ‖ Fat **10g**, Carb **43g**, Protein **9g**, Fiber **8g**, Calories **284**
Cook Time: 5 mins, **Total Time**: 5 mins, **Servings**: 2
Yield: 2 servings

Ingredients

2 tablespoons of natural nut butter, such as almond, cashew or peanut
1 teaspoon of honey
A pinch of salt
1 whole-wheat bagel, split and toasted
1 small banana, sliced

Directions

In a small bowl, mix nut butter, honey and salt. Put the mixture on the bagel halves and add banana slices on top.

Crunchy Roasted Chickpeas

Nutrition Facts || Fat **2g**, Carb **17g**, Protein **6g**, Fiber **5g**, Calories **100**
Active Time: 5 mins, **Additional Time**: 30 mins
Total Time: 35 mins, **Servings**: 4
Yield: 4 servings

Ingredients
1 (15 ounce) can of no-salt-added chickpeas, rinsed
Nonstick cooking spray
¼ teaspoon of sea salt

Directions
Heat the oven to 425°F. Dry the chickpeas with paper towels and put them on a large baking sheet with edges. Spray with cooking spray and add salt. Bake until they are crunchy, 30 to 45 minutes.

Banana & Walnuts

Nutrition Facts ‖ Fat **13g**, Carb **30g**, Protein **4g**, Fiber **4g**, Calories **236**
Prep Time: 5 mins, **Total Time**: 5 mins, **Servings**: 1
Yield: 1 servings

Ingredients
10 walnut halves
1 medium banana

Directions
Put the walnuts in a small bowl or a container that you can take with you. Have the banana with the walnuts as a snack.

Diabetes-friendly Recipes

- Chicken Kebabs with Warm Cabbage-Apple Slaw & Potatoes
- Lentil Stew with Salsa Verde
- One-Pot Garlicky Shrimp & Spinach
- Roasted Salmon with Smoky Chickpeas & Greens
- Slow-Cooked Ranch Chicken and Vegetables
- Spaghetti Squash with Roasted Tomatoes, Beans & Almond Pesto
- Chicken, Potato, and Gravy Bowls
- Beer-Battered Fish Tacos with Tomato & Avocado Salsa
- Sheet-Pan Chili-Lime Salmon with Potatoes & Peppers
- Four-Bean & Pumpkin Chili
- Slow-Cooker Chicken Marsala
- Provençal Baked Fish with Roasted Potatoes & Mushrooms

Chicken Kebabs with Warm Cabbage-Apple Slaw & Potatoes

Nutrition Facts || Fat **16g**, Carb **37g**, Protein **41g**, Fiber **6g**, Calories **452**
Active Time: 45 mins, **Additional Time**: 1 hr
Total Time: 1hr 45 mins, **Servings**: 4
Yield: 4 servings

Ingredients

1 orange
¼ cup of finely chopped onion
2 tablespoons of coarse ground mustard
2 teaspoons of grated fresh ginger
½ teaspoon of salt, divided
½ teaspoon of ground pepper, divided
1 ½ pounds of boneless, skinless chicken breasts, cut into 1 ½-inch pieces
1 ½ pounds of round red or yellow potatoes
2 cloves of garlic, thinly sliced
2 tablespoons of extra-virgin olive oil
3 cups of warm cabbage-apple slaw

Directions

Grate and squeeze orange. In a small bowl, mix 1/3 cup of the orange juice, ½ tsp. of the orange zest, onion, mustard, ginger, and ¼ teaspoon each of salt and pepper. Put chicken in a plastic bag that can be sealed and place it in a shallow dish. Pour the marinade over the chicken. Seal the bag and turn it to coat the chicken. Keep it in the fridge for 1 to 3 hours, turning once or twice.

Meanwhile, Make two 18-by-12-inch rectangles by folding two 24-by-18-inch pieces of heavy foil in half.

Cut potatoes into 1-inch pieces. Split the potatoes and garlic between the foil rectangles. Drizzle with oil and add the remaining ¼ teaspoon each of salt and pepper.

For each packet, bring up two opposite sides of foil and seal them with a double fold. Fold the other sides to close the potato mixture, leaving room for steam to build.

Heat the grill to medium.

Cover and grill the packets for 15 minutes. Turn the potatoes to avoid burning.

After the potatoes have been grilling for 15 minutes, take out the chicken and throw away the marinade. Put the chicken on nine 6- to 8-inch skewers, place on grill rack, and close grill cover. Grill the kebabs, turning once, until the chicken is done, about 15 minutes. Keep grilling the potatoes, turning every 10-15 minutes until the potatoes are soft, about 10 to 15 minutes more.

Take the potato packets off the grill and open them carefully. Serve the kebabs with slaw and potatoes.

Lentil Stew with Salsa Verde

Nutrition Facts || Fat **5g**, Carb **53g**, Protein **19g**, Fiber **14g**, Calories **322**
Prep Time: 30 mins, **Additional Time**: 10 mins
Total Time: 40 mins, **Servings**: 4
Yield: 4 servings

Ingredients

1 tablespoon of olive oil

1 ¼ cups of finely chopped celery (4-6 stalks) or fennel (1 bulb)

3 small carrots, peeled and finely chopped (1/2 cup)

½ cup of finely chopped red bell pepper

5 tablespoons of finely chopped shallot (1 large), divided

2 large cloves of garlic, minced

2 tablespoons of tomato paste

1 ½ cups of French green lentils, sorted and rinsed

4 cups of low-sodium chicken broth or vegetable broth, or water

¾ teaspoon of ground pepper, divided

½ teaspoon of salt, divided

1 small bunch of Italian parsley, finely chopped (about ¾ cup)

1 large lime, juiced (2 Tbsp.)

2 tablespoons of white-wine vinegar

Directions

In a 4- to 6-qt. pot, heat oil over medium-high heat. Add celery (or fennel), carrots, bell pepper, 3 Tbsp. shallot, and garlic and cook, stirring, until they are soft, about 3 minutes. Stir in tomato paste and cook for another 30 seconds. Add lentils, broth (or water), ½ tsp. pepper, and ¼ tsp. salt and bring to a boil. Cover, lower the heat, and simmer until the lentils are done, 35 to 40 minutes.

While the stew is cooking, make the salsa verde by mixing parsley, lime juice, vinegar, and the remaining 2 Tbsp. shallot and ¼ tsp. each of pepper and salt in a small bowl.

To serve, put the stew in 4 bowls and add some salsa verde on top of each. Serve the rest of the salsa verde on the side.

Tips
You can make the stew up to Step 1 and keep it in the fridge for up to 3 days. Reheat it on the stove or in the microwave, adding water if needed.

One-Pot Garlicky Shrimp & Spinach

Nutrition Facts || Fat **12g**, Carb **6g**, Protein **26g**, Fiber **3g**, Calories **226**
Active Time: 25 mins, **Total Time**: 25 mins, **Servings**: 4
Yield: 4 cups

Ingredients

3 tablespoons of extra-virgin olive oil, divided
6 medium cloves of garlic, sliced, divided
1 pound of spinach
¼ teaspoon of salt plus 1/8 teaspoon, divided
1 tablespoon of lemon juice
1 pound of shrimp (21-30 count), peeled and deveined
¼ teaspoon of crushed red pepper
1 tablespoon of finely chopped fresh parsley
1 ½ teaspoons of lemon zest

Directions

In a large pot, heat 1 tablespoon of oil over medium heat. Cook half of the garlic until it starts to brown, 1 to 2 minutes. Add spinach and ¼ teaspoon of salt and toss well. Cook, stirring once or twice, until the spinach is mostly wilted, 3 to 5 minutes. Take off the heat and stir in lemon juice. Put in a bowl and keep warm.

Turn up the heat to medium-high and add the remaining 2 tablespoons of oil to the same pot. Cook the rest of the garlic until it starts to brown, 1 to 2 minutes. Add shrimp, red pepper flakes and the remaining 1/8 teaspoon of salt and cook, stirring, until the shrimp are done, 3 to 5 minutes more. Put the shrimp on top of the spinach and sprinkle with lemon zest and parsley.

Roasted Salmon with Smoky Chickpeas & Greens

Nutrition Facts ‖ Fat **22g**, Carb **23g**, Protein **37g**, Fiber **6g**, Calories **447**
Prep Time: 40 mins, **Total Time**: 40 mins, **Servings**: 4
Yield: 4 servings

Ingredients

2 tablespoons of extra-virgin olive oil, divided
1 tablespoon of smoked paprika
½ teaspoon of salt, divided, plus a pinch
1 (15 ounce) can of no-salt-added chickpeas, rinsed
⅓ cup of buttermilk
¼ cup of mayonnaise
¼ cup of chopped fresh chives and/or dill, plus more for garnish
½ teaspoon of ground pepper, divided
¼ teaspoon of garlic powder
10 cups of chopped kale
¼ cup of water
1 ¼ pounds of wild salmon, cut into 4 portions

Directions

Heat the oven to 425 degrees F and arrange the racks in the upper third and middle. In a medium bowl, toss chickpeas with 1 tablespoon oil, paprika and ¼ teaspoon salt after patting them very dry. Put them on a baking sheet with edges and bake on the upper rack, stirring twice, for 30 minutes.

In the meantime, blend buttermilk, mayonnaise, herbs, ¼ teaspoon pepper and garlic powder in a blender until smooth. Keep it aside.

In a large skillet, heat the remaining 1 tablespoon of oil over medium heat. Add kale and stir occasionally for 2 minutes. Add water and keep stirring until the kale is soft, about 5 minutes more. Take it off the heat and add a pinch of salt.

Take the chickpeas out of the oven and move them to one side of the pan. Put salmon on the other side and sprinkle with the remaining ¼ teaspoon each salt and pepper. Bake until the salmon is done, 5 to 8 minutes.

Pour the dressing you kept aside on the salmon, add more herbs if you like, and serve with the kale and chickpeas.

Slow-Cooked Ranch Chicken and Vegetables

Nutrition Facts || Fat **10g**, Carb **21g**, Protein **31g**, Fiber **4g**, Calories **291**
Prep Time: 30 mins, **Additional Time**: 6 hrs 45 mins
Total Time: 7 hrs 15 mins, **Servings**: 6
Yield: 6 servings

Ingredients

2 medium onions, cut into thin wedges

1 tablespoon of dried minced onion

2 teaspoons of dried parsley flakes, crushed

1 teaspoon of garlic powder

1 teaspoon of salt

1 teaspoon of black pepper

½ teaspoon of dried thyme, crushed

½ teaspoon of dried dill

5 pounds of large chicken thighs, skinned (12 to 14 total)

2 (10.75 ounce) cans of reduced-fat, reduced-sodium condensed cream of chicken soup

1 (8 ounce) carton of sour cream

2 to 3 teaspoons of finely chopped canned chipotle chile peppers in adobo sauce

2 medium red and/or green sweet peppers, cut into ½-inch-thick strips

2 medium zucchini, halved lengthwise and thinly sliced

1 3-pound of spaghetti squash

¼ cup of snipped fresh parsley (Optional)

Directions

Put onion wedges in a slow cooker that can hold 5 to 6 quarts. Mix dried onion, parsley flakes, garlic powder, salt, black pepper, thyme, and dill in a small bowl. Layer one-third of the chicken thighs over the onions in the slow cooker in a single layer. Sprinkle about one-third of the spice mix over the chicken. Do this two more times with the remaining chicken thighs and spice mix.

In a medium bowl, mix condensed soup, sour cream, and chile peppers. Pour over the chicken in the slow cooker.

Cover and cook on low-heat for 6 to 7 hours or on high-heat for 3 to 3 ½ hours. If using low-heat, switch to high-heat. Add sweet pepper strips and squash slices to the slow cooker. Cover and cook for another 45 minutes.

Meanwhile, cut spaghetti squash in half lengthwise and remove seeds and strings. Put one half, cut side down, in a dish that can go in the microwave. Prick the skin all over with a fork. Microwave on high for 10 to 12 minutes or until you can easily pierce it with a fork; take it out of the dish carefully. Do the same with the other squash half. Let the squash cool a bit. Use a fork to pull and separate the squash flesh into strands.

Take all of the chicken thighs out of the slow cooker (see Tips). Put 6 of the thighs on a plate and cover with foil to keep them warm. Let the sauce and vegetables in the slow cooker cool a bit (the sauce will get thicker as it cools). While the sauce cools, take the meat off the remaining chicken thighs. Use two forks to shred the meat. Throw away the bones. Put the shredded chicken in a very large bowl and set it aside.

To serve, put spaghetti squash on six plates. Put one of the whole chicken thighs on top of the squash on each plate. Stir the sauce and vegetable mixture in the slow cooker. Spoon about ½ cup of the sauce and vegetable mixture over each serving. Sprinkle with fresh parsley if you want.

Mix the rest of the sauce and vegetable mixture from the slow cooker with the shredded chicken in the bowl. Cover and keep in the fridge for up to 2 days; use it to make Chipotle Ranch Chicken Pasta (see associated recipe), if you want.

Tips

Chile peppers have oils that can burn your skin and eyes, so try not to touch them too much. When you work with chile peppers, wear plastic or rubber gloves. If you touch the peppers with your bare hands, wash your hands and nails well with soap and warm water.

Make sure you check the sauce and vegetable mixture for any chicken bones that may have come off the meat while cooking or taking out the chicken.

The extra shredded chicken from this recipe can be used for another meal. Cover and keep the extra chicken (Step 7) in the fridge for up to 2 days.

Spaghetti Squash with Roasted Tomatoes, Beans & Almond Pesto

Nutrition Facts || Fat **26g**, Carb **37g**, Protein **12g**, Fiber **10g**, Calories **400**
Prep Time: 45 mins, **Total Time**: 45 mins, **Servings**: 4
Yield: 4 servings

Ingredients
Almond Pesto:
2 cups of fresh basil leaves
1 cup of fresh parsley leaves
½ cup of grated Parmesan cheese
⅓ cup of whole raw almonds
1 clove of garlic
1 ½ tablespoons of red-wine vinegar
¼ teaspoon of kosher salt
¼ teaspoon of ground pepper
¼ cup of extra-virgin olive oil
¼ cup of water

Spaghetti Squash & Vegetables:
1 3-pound of spaghetti squash
¼ cup of water
2 pints of grape tomatoes, halved
1 tablespoon of extra-virgin olive oil
¼ teaspoon of kosher salt
¼ teaspoon of ground pepper
1 cup of canned cannellini beans, rinsed

Directions
For the pesto: Put basil, parsley, Parmesan, almonds, garlic, vinegar and ¼
teaspoon each salt and pepper in a food processor and pulse until coarsely chopped,

scraping down the sides. While the motor is running, pour in ¼ cup oil; process until well mixed.

To the pesto in the food processor, add water and pulse to combine.

For the squash and vegetables: Heat oven to 400 degrees F. Cover a baking sheet with edges with foil.

Cut squash in half lengthwise and remove the seeds. Put cut-side down in a dish that can go in the microwave and add water. Microwave on High until you can easily scrape the flesh with a fork, about 15 minutes.

In the meantime, mix tomatoes with oil, salt and pepper in a large bowl. Put on the prepared baking sheet. Roast until soft and wrinkled, 10 to 12 minutes. Take out of the oven. Add beans and stir to combine.

Pull the squash flesh into the bowl and split among 4 plates. Put some of the tomato-bean mixture and about 3 tablespoons pesto sauce on each portion.

Tips
You can keep pesto (Step 1) in the fridge for up to 5 days.

You can use leftovers to make a pesto-turkey sandwich for lunch; Spread 1 ½ Tbsp. leftover pesto on 2 slices toasted whole-wheat bread. Add 3 oz. sliced deli turkey, 2 lettuce leaves and 2 tomato slices.

Chicken, Potato, and Gravy Bowls

Nutrition Facts || Fat **9g**, Carb **35g**, Protein **22g**, Fiber **4g**, Calories **312**
Prep Time: 15 mins, **Additional Time**: 35 mins
Total Time: 50 mins, **Servings**: 4
Yield: 4 servings

Ingredients

1 ½ pounds of Yukon gold potatoes or other potatoes, quartered
1 tablespoon of canola oil
12 ounces of skinless boneless chicken thighs
2 teaspoons of bottled minced roasted garlic
¼ cup of light sour cream
¼ cup of fat free milk
2 teaspoons of snipped fresh thyme or Italian (flat-leaf) parsley
¼ teaspoon of salt
⅛ teaspoon of ground black pepper
1 (.87 ounce) package of 30 percent less sodium brown gravy mix
1 Sprig of fresh thyme or Italian parsley

Directions

Boil potatoes in a large pot with a little water, covered, for 20 to 25 minutes or until soft. While the potatoes are cooking, heat oil in a large skillet over medium-high heat. Turn down the heat to medium and add chicken thighs. Cook for 14 to 18 minutes, or until cooked through, flipping once halfway through. Pull the chicken apart into chunks. Cover and keep warm.

Pour out the water from the cooked potatoes and put them back in the pot. Add garlic to the potatoes. Use a potato masher or an electric mixer on low speed to mash them. Add sour cream, milk, 2 teaspoons thyme, salt, and pepper. Mash until smooth and fluffy. Cover with foil and keep warm. Make gravy according to the package directions. To serve, put potatoes in bowls, then chicken, and pour gravy over them. If you want, put a thyme sprig on each serving.

Sheet-Pan Chili-Lime Salmon with Potatoes & Peppers

Nutrition Facts || Fat **17g**, Carb **26g**, Protein **35g**, Fiber **3g**, Calories **405**
Prep Time: 25 mins, **Total Time**: 25 mins, **Servings**: 4
Yield: 1 serving

Ingredients

1 pound of Yukon Gold potatoes, cut into ¾-inch pieces

2 tablespoons of extra-virgin olive oil, divided

¾ teaspoon of salt, divided

¼ teaspoon of ground pepper

2 teaspoons of chili powder

1 teaspoon of ground cumin

½ teaspoon of garlic powder

1 lime, zested and quartered

2 medium bell peppers, any color, sliced

1 ¼ pounds of center-cut salmon fillet, skinned, if desired, and cut into 4 portions

Directions

Heat the oven to 425 degrees F and spray a large baking sheet with edges with cooking spray. Mix potatoes, 1 tablespoon oil, ¼ teaspoon salt and pepper in a medium bowl. Put them on the prepared pan and bake for 15 minutes.

In the meantime, mix chili powder, cumin, garlic powder, lime zest and the remaining ½ teaspoon salt in a small bowl. Put bell peppers in the medium bowl and add the remaining 1 tablespoon oil and ½ tablespoon of the spice mix; toss well to coat. Coat the salmon with the rest of the spice mix.

After 15 minutes, take the pan out of the oven. Add the peppers and toss to combine. Bake for 5 minutes. Take out of the oven; move some of the vegetables aside and put the salmon on the pan. Bake until the salmon is done, 6 to 8 minutes. Serve with lime wedges.

Four-Bean & Pumpkin Chili

Nutrition Facts || Fat **3g**, Carb **49g**, Protein **14g**, Fiber **17g**, Calories **276**
Prep Time: 45 mins, **Additional Time**: 40 mins
Total Time: 1hr 25 mins, **Servings**: 8
Yield: 8 servings

Ingredients

1 tablespoon of extra-virgin olive oil

3 cups of chopped onion

1 ½ cups of chopped carrot

3 large cloves of garlic, minced

4 cups of low-sodium vegetable broth

3 cups of diced pumpkin or butternut squash

1 (28 ounce) can of no-salt-added crushed tomatoes

4 (15 ounce) cans of low-sodium beans, such as black, great northern, pinto and/or red, rinsed

3 tablespoons of chili powder

2 teaspoons of ground cumin

1 teaspoon of ground cinnamon

¾ teaspoon of salt

¼ teaspoon of cayenne pepper

Diced onion, sliced jalapeños, Cotija cheese and/or pepitas for garnish

Directions

In a large pot, heat oil over medium-high heat. Add onion and cook, stirring often, until it begins to brown, about 5 minutes. Lower the heat to medium, add carrot and keep cooking, stirring often, until the vegetables are soft, 4 to 5 minutes more. Add garlic and cook, stirring, for 1 minute.

Add broth, scraping up any browned bits, and let it boil over high heat. Add pumpkin (or squash), tomatoes, beans, chili powder, cumin, cinnamon, salt and cayenne (if using). Cover and bring it back to a boil. Lower the heat to keep a gentle simmer and cook, uncovered, until the pumpkin (or squash) is soft, about 30 minutes.

Top with onion, jalapeños, cheese and/or pepitas, if you like, and serve.

Tips
You can keep in the fridge for up to 5 days; freeze up to 6 months.

Slow-Cooker Chicken Marsala

Nutrition Facts || Fat **6g**, Carb **57g**, Protein **47g**, Fiber **6g**, Calories **479**
Prep Time: 20 mins, **Additional Time**: 3 hrs 30 mins
Total Time: 3 hrs 50 mins, **Servings**: 4
Yield: 4 servings

Ingredients

3 tablespoons of all-purpose flour

1 cup of low-sodium chicken broth, divided

12 ounces of cremini mushrooms, stemmed and thinly sliced (about 4 cups)

½ cup of chopped shallots

⅓ cup of dry Marsala

1 tablespoon of chopped fresh thyme

4 (6 ounce) of boneless, skinless chicken breasts

¾ teaspoon of salt

½ teaspoon of ground pepper

8 ounces of whole-wheat spaghetti

2 tablespoons of chopped fresh flat-leaf parsley

Directions

In a small bowl, whisk flour and ½ cup broth until smooth. In a 6-quart slow cooker, mix the flour mixture, mushrooms, shallots, Marsala, thyme and the remaining ½ cup broth. Put chicken in one layer in the slow cooker and season with salt and pepper. Cover and cook on Low until a thermometer in the thickest part of the chicken shows 165 degrees F, 3 hours to 3 hours 30 minutes.

Boil pasta as the package says; drain. Put the chicken on the pasta. Pour the Marsala sauce over it and sprinkle with parsley.

Provençal Baked Fish with Roasted Potatoes & Mushrooms

Nutrition Facts || Fat **9g**, Carb **25g**, Protein **24g**, Fiber **3g**, Calories **276**
Prep Time: 15 mins, **Additional Time**: 45 mins
Total Time: 1hr, **Servings**: 4
Yield: 4 servings

Ingredients

1 pound of Yukon Gold or red potatoes, cubed
1 pound of mushrooms (shiitake, cremini, oyster or other fresh mushrooms), trimmed and sliced
2 tablespoons of extra-virgin olive oil, divided
¼ teaspoon of salt
¼ teaspoon of ground pepper
2 cloves of garlic, peeled and sliced
14 ounces of halibut, grouper or cod fillet, cut into 4 portions
4 tablespoons of lemon juice
1 teaspoon of herbes de Provence
Fresh thyme for garnish

Directions

Heat the oven to 425 degrees F.

In a large bowl, mix potatoes, mushrooms, 1 Tbsp. oil, salt, and pepper. Put them in a 9x13-inch baking dish. Bake until the vegetables are tender, 30 to 40 minutes.

Stir the vegetables and add garlic. Put fish on top. Pour lemon juice and the remaining 1 Tbsp. oil over it. Sprinkle with herbes de Provence. Bake until the fish is cooked through and breaks easily, 10 to 15 minutes. If you want, put thyme on top.

Vegan & Vegetarian Recipes

- Vegan Smoothie Bowl
- Meal-Prep Vegan Lettuce Wraps
- Vegan Superfood Grain Bowl
- Spinach-Avocado smoothie
- Chickpea & Roasted Red Pepper Lettuce Wraps with Tahini Dressing
- Chickpea & Quinoa Grain Bowl
- Vegetarian Stuffed Cabbage
- Falafel Burgers
- Veggie & Hummus Sandwich

Vegan Smoothie Bowl

Nutrition Facts || Fat **10g**, Carb **64g**, Protein **9g**, Fiber **12g**, Calories **338**
Prep Time: 10 mins, **Total Time**: 10 mins, **Servings**: 1
Yield: 1 serving

Ingredients

1 large banana
1 cup of frozen mixed berries
½ cup of unsweetened soymilk or other unsweetened non-dairy milk
¼ cup of pineapple chunks
½ kiwi, sliced
1 tablespoon of sliced almonds, toasted if desired
1 tablespoon of unsweetened coconut flakes, toasted if desired
1 teaspoon of chia seeds

Directions

Put banana, berries and soymilk (or almond milk) in a blender and blend until smooth.

Put the smoothie in a bowl and add pineapple, kiwi, almonds, coconut and chia seeds on top.

Meal-Prep Vegan Lettuce Wraps

Nutrition Facts || Fat **20g**, Carb **50g**, Protein **14g**, Fiber **14g**, Calories **425**
Prep Time: 10 mins, **Total Time**: 10 mins, **Servings**: 4
Yield: 4 containers

Ingredients

2 heads of butter or Bibb lettuce, leaves separated
1 ½ cups of cooked quinoa, cooled to room temperature
4 cups of Bean Salad with Lemon-Cumin Dressing
⅓ cup of chopped fresh mint (reserved from bean salad recipe)

Directions

For 1 serving of lettuce wraps: Put 3 lettuce leaves in a container with a lid. Add 2 tablespoons quinoa and 1/3 cup bean salad on each leaf. Sprinkle 1 ½ teaspoons mint on each one. Keep in the fridge for up to 1 day.

Tips

You can keep cooked quinoa in the fridge for up to 4 days or freeze it for up to 3 months. The bean salad can stay in the fridge for up to 4 days (don't add the mint until you make the wraps).

Vegan Superfood Grain Bowls

Nutrition Facts ‖ Fat **19g**, Carb **43g**, Protein **16g**, Fiber **13g**, Calories **381**
Active Time: 15 mins, **Total Time**: 15 mins, **Servings**: 4
Yield: 4 containers

Ingredients

1 (8 ounce) of pouch microwavable quinoa
½ cup of hummus
2 tablespoons of lemon juice
1 (5 ounce) of packaged baby kale
1 (8 ounce) of packaged refrigerated cooked whole baby beets, sliced (or 2 cups from salad bar)
1 cup of frozen shelled edamame, thawed
1 medium avocado, sliced
¼ cup of unsalted toasted sunflower seeds

Directions

Cook quinoa as the package says; let it cool down.

Mix hummus and lemon juice in a small bowl. Add water to make it as thin as you want for a dressing. Put the dressing in 4 small containers with lids and keep in the fridge.

Put baby kale in 4 containers with lids. Add ½ cup quinoa, 1/2 cup beets, 1/4 cup edamame and 1 tablespoon sunflower seeds on each one.

When you want to eat, add 1/4 avocado and the hummus dressing on top.

Spinach-Avocado Smoothie

Nutrition Facts || Fat **8g**, Carb **58g**, Protein **18g**, Fiber **8g**, Calories **357**
Prep Time: 5 mins, **Total Time**: 5 mins, **Servings**: 1
Yield: 2 cups

Ingredients

1 cup of nonfat plain yogurt
1 cup of fresh spinach
1 frozen banana
¼ avocado
2 tablespoons of water
1 teaspoon of honey

Directions

Put yogurt, spinach, banana, avocado, water and honey in a blender and blend until smooth.

Chickpea & Roasted Red Pepper Lettuce Wraps with Tahini Dressing

Nutrition Facts || Fat **28g**, Carb **44g**, Protein **16g**, Fiber **10g**, Calories **498**
Prep Time: 10 mins, **Total Time**: 10 mins, **Servings**: 4
Yield: 12 wraps

Ingredients
¼ cup of tahini
¼ cup of extra-virgin olive oil
1 teaspoon of lemon zest
¼ cup of lemon juice (from 2 lemons)
1 ½ teaspoons of pure maple syrup
¾ teaspoon of kosher salt
½ teaspoon of paprika
2 (15 ounce) cans of no-salt-added chickpeas, rinsed
½ cup of sliced jarred roasted red peppers, drained
½ cup of thinly sliced shallots
12 large Bibb of lettuce leaves
¼ cup of toasted almonds, chopped
2 tablespoons of chopped fresh parsley

Directions
In a large bowl, whisk tahini, oil, lemon zest, lemon juice, maple syrup, salt and paprika. Add chickpeas, peppers and shallots and toss to coat them.

Put some of the mixture on each lettuce leaf (about 1/3 cup per leaf). Sprinkle almonds and parsley on top. Fold the lettuce leaves around the filling and enjoy.

Chickpea & Quinoa Grain Bowl

Nutrition Facts || Fat **17g**, Carb **75g**, Protein **18g**, Fiber **16g**, Calories **503**
Prep Time: 15 mins, **Total Time**: 15 mins, **Servings**: 1
Yield: 1 serving

Ingredients

1 cup of cooked quinoa
⅓ cup of canned chickpeas, rinsed and drained
½ cup of cucumber slices
½ cup of cherry tomatoes, halved
¼ avocado, diced
3 tablespoons of hummus
1 tablespoon of finely chopped roasted red pepper
1 tablespoon of lemon juice
1 tablespoon of water, plus more if desired
1 teaspoon of chopped fresh parsley (Optional)
A pinch of salt
A pinch of ground pepper

Directions

Put quinoa, chickpeas, cucumbers, tomatoes and avocado in a big bowl.

Mix hummus, roasted red pepper, lemon juice and water in a bowl. Add more water to make the dressing as thin as you like. Add parsley, salt and pepper and mix well. Have it with the Buddha bowl.

Vegetarian Stuffed Cabbage

Nutrition Facts || Fat **24g**, Carb **61g**, Protein **14g**, Fiber **12g**, Calories **544**
Cook Time: 1 hr 15 mins, **Additional Time**: 45 mins
Total Time: 2hrs, **Servings**: 4
Yield: 4 servings

Ingredients

1 cup of water

½ cup of short-grain brown rice

1 teaspoon of extra-virgin olive oil plus 2 tablespoons, divided

1 large Savoy cabbage (2-3 pounds)

1 pound of baby bella mushrooms, finely chopped

1 large onion, finely chopped

4 cloves of garlic, minced

½ teaspoon of dried rubbed sage

½ teaspoon of crumbled dried rosemary

½ teaspoon of salt, divided

¼ teaspoon of freshly ground pepper plus 1/8 teaspoon, divided

½ cup of red wine

¼ cup of dried currants

1/3 cup of toasted pine nuts, chopped

2 tablespoons of extra-virgin olive oil, divided

1 small onion, chopped

Garlic, minced

¼ teaspoon of salt

¼ teaspoon of freshly ground pepper

1 28-ounce can of no-salt-added crushed tomatoes

½ cup red wine

Directions

To make cabbage and filling: In a medium saucepan, bring water, rice and 1 teaspoon oil to a boil. Lower the heat to keep a very low simmer, cover and cook until the water is absorbed and the rice is tender, 40 to 50 minutes. Put in a large bowl and set aside.

At the same time, fill a large pot halfway with water and bring to a boil. Put a clean kitchen towel on a baking sheet and place it near the stove.

With a small, sharp knife, cut out the core from the bottom of the cabbage. Put the cabbage in the boiling water and cook for 5 minutes. As the leaves get soft, use tongs to gently take out 8 large outer leaves. Put the leaves on the baking sheet and pat them dry with more towels. Set aside.

Let the rest of the cabbage drain in a colander for a few minutes. Chop enough to get about 3 cups. (Keep any remaining cabbage for something else.)

Heat 1 ½ tablespoons oil in a large skillet over medium-high heat. Add mushrooms, onion, garlic, sage, rosemary and ¼ teaspoon each salt and pepper; cook, stirring, until the mushrooms have given off their juices and the pan is fairly dry, 8 to 10 minutes. Add wine and cook, stirring, until it's gone, about 3 minutes more. Add the mixture to the cooked rice along with currants and pine nuts.

In the skillet over medium-high heat, heat the remaining ½ tablespoon oil. Add the chopped cabbage, the remaining ¼ teaspoon salt and 1/8 teaspoon pepper; cook, stirring, until the cabbage is wilted and starting to brown, 3 to 5 minutes. Add to the rice mixture.

To make sauce: Heat 1 tablespoon oil in a large skillet over medium heat. Add onion, garlic, salt and pepper and cook, stirring, until they start to soften, 2 to 4 minutes. Add tomatoes and wine; bring to a simmer and cook until slightly thicker, about 10 minutes.

Heat oven to 375 degrees F.

To stuff cabbage: Put a reserved cabbage leaf on your work surface; cut out the thick stem in the middle, keeping the leaf whole. Put about ¾ cup filling in the middle. Fold both sides over the filling and roll up. Do the same with the remaining 7 leaves and filling.

Spread 1 cup of the tomato sauce in a 9-by-13-inch baking dish. Put the stuffed cabbage rolls, seam side down, on the sauce. Pour the rest of the sauce over the rolls and drizzle with the remaining 1 tablespoon oil.

Bake while uncovered, until hot, about 45 minutes, basting twice with the sauce

Tips

You can make it up to Step 10, cover and keep in the fridge for up to 1 day. Let it sit at room temperature for about 30 minutes before baking.

For the Best Flavor: Toast nuts and seeds before using them in a recipe. To toast small nuts, chopped nuts & seeds, put them in a small dry skillet and cook over medium-low heat, stirring constantly, until they smell good and are lightly browned, 2 to 4 minutes.

Sodium Variation: Sodium levels vary a lot among brands of plum and crushed. And even though it can be hard to find any that say "no-salt-added," we use brands that have little or no added sodium for the best tomato flavor. Look at nutrition labels and choose one that has 190 mg sodium or less per ½-cup serving.

Falafel Burgers

Nutrition Facts || Fat **7g**, Carb **43g**, Protein **10g**, Fiber **8g**, Calories **267**
Prep Time: 30 mins, **Additional Time**: 30 mins
Total Time:1hr, **Servings**: 4
Yield: 4 servings

Ingredients

½ cup of coarsely chopped onion

3 cloves of garlic, crushed

1 medium jalapeño pepper, seeded and coarsely chopped

¾ cup of fresh cilantro and/or parsley leaves

1 (15 ounce) can of no-salt-added chickpeas, rinsed

2 teaspoons of ground cumin

1 teaspoon of ground coriander

¼ teaspoon of baking soda

¼ teaspoon of salt

⅓ cup of dry whole-wheat breadcrumbs or gluten-free breadcrumbs

1 tablespoon of extra-virgin olive oil

4 whole-wheat or gluten-free burger buns, split and toasted

Directions

Put onion, garlic, jalapeño and cilantro (or parsley) in a food processor and pulse until they are chopped evenly. Add chickpeas, cumin, coriander, baking soda and salt. Process until well mixed. Put in a medium bowl. Add breadcrumbs. Cover and keep in the fridge for 20 minutes. (This lets the breadcrumbs soak up extra moisture.)

Heat the oven to 375 degrees F. Make four 3-inch-diameter patties with about 1/3 cup of the chickpea mixture for each patty.

In a large skillet, heat oil over medium heat. Cook the patties until golden and crispy, about 4 minutes per side. Move the patties to a baking sheet carefully; bake until warm and slightly puffy, about 15 minutes. Have the patties on buns.

Veggie & Hummus Sandwich

Nutrition Facts || Fat **14g**, Carb **40g**, Protein **13g**, Fiber **12g**, Calories **325**
Active Time: 10 mins, **Total Time**: 10 mins, **Servings**: 1
Yield: 1 sandwich

Ingredients

2 slices of whole-grain bread

3 tablespoons of hummus

¼ avocado, mashed

½ cup of mixed salad greens

¼ medium red bell pepper, sliced

¼ cup of sliced cucumber

¼ cup of shredded carrot

Directions

Put hummus on one slice of bread and avocado on the other. Add greens, bell pepper, cucumber and carrot to the sandwich. Cut it in half and enjoy.

Special Seasonal Recipes

- Summer Skillet Vegetable & Egg Scramble
- Pumpkin Pie Smoothie
- Oatmeal-Rhubarb Porridge
- Pumpkin Overnight Oats
- Slow-Cooker Pasta e Fagioli Soup
- Winter Vegetable Mulligatawny Soup
- Lemony Linguine with Spring Vegetables
- Winter Kale & Quinoa Salad with Avocado

Summer Skillet Vegetable & Egg Scramble

Nutrition Facts || Fat **14g**, Carb **20g**, Protein **12g**, Fiber **4g**, Calories **254**
Prep Time: 30 mins, **Total Time**: 30 mins, **Servings**: 4
Yield: 6 cups

Ingredients

2 tablespoons of olive oil

12 ounces of baby potatoes, thinly sliced

4 cups of thinly sliced vegetables, such as mushrooms, bell peppers, and/or zucchini (14 oz.)

3 scallions, thinly sliced, green and white parts separated

1 teaspoon of minced fresh herbs, such as rosemary or thyme

6 large eggs (or 4 large eggs plus 4 egg whites), lightly beaten

2 cups of packed leafy greens, such as baby spinach or baby kale (2 oz.)

½ teaspoon of salt

Directions

In a large skillet that is cast-iron or nonstick, heat oil over medium heat. Put potatoes in and cook, stirring a few times, until they start to soften, about 8 minutes.

Put sliced vegetables and scallion whites in and cook without a cover, stirring sometimes, until the vegetables are soft and lightly browned, 8 to 10 minutes. Stir in herbs. Move the vegetable mixture to the edge of the pan.

Turn down the heat to medium-low. Put eggs and scallion greens in the middle of the pan. Cook, stirring, until the eggs are softly scrambled, about 2 minutes.

Mix leafy greens with the eggs. Take off the heat and stir to combine well. Stir in salt.

Pumpkin Pie Smoothie

Nutrition Facts ‖ Fat **6g**, Carb **42g**, Protein **10g**, Fiber **6g**, Calories **247**
Prep Time: 5 mins, **Total Time**: 5 mins, **Servings**: 1
Yield: 1 smoothie

Ingredients

1 medium frozen banana
½ cup of unsweetened almond milk or other nut milk
⅓ cup of plain whole-milk Greek yogurt
⅓ cup of canned pumpkin puree
⅛ teaspoon of pumpkin pie spice
1-2 teaspoons of pure maple syrup

Directions

Put banana, almond milk (or other nut milk), yogurt, pumpkin puree, pumpkin pie spice and maple syrup in a blender and blend until smooth.

Oatmeal-Rhubarb Porridge

Nutrition Facts || Fat **8g**, Carb **56g**, Protein **13g**, Fiber **6g**, Calories **336**
Cook Time: 20 mins, **Total Time**: 20 mins, **Servings**: 2
Yield: 2 servings

Ingredients

1 ½ cups of nonfat milk or nondairy milk, such as soymilk or almond milk

½ cup of orange juice

1 cup of old-fashioned rolled oats

1 cup of ½-inch pieces rhubarb, fresh or frozen

½ teaspoon of ground cinnamon

A pinch of salt

2-3 tablespoons of brown sugar, pure maple syrup or agave syrup

2 tablespoons of chopped pecans or other nuts, toasted, if desired

Directions

In a medium saucepan, mix milk, juice, oats, rhubarb, cinnamon and salt. Bring to a boil over medium-high heat. Lower the heat, cover and cook at a very low boil, stirring often, until the oats and rhubarb are soft, about 5 minutes. Take off the heat and let sit, covered, for 5 minutes. Add sweetener as you like. Sprinkle with nuts.

Tips

To make chopped nuts toasted, put them in a small dry skillet and cook over medium-low heat, stirring all the time, until they smell good and are lightly browned, 2 to 4 minutes.

Oats that are labeled "gluten-free" should be used by people who have celiac disease or gluten-sensitivity, as wheat and barley often cross-contaminate oats.

Pumpkin Overnight Oats

Nutrition Facts ‖ Fat **4g**, Carb **41g**, Protein **6g**, Fiber **6g**, Calories **218**
Prep Time: 10 mins, **Additional Time**: 7 hrs 50 mins
Total Time: 8hrs, **Servings**: 1
Yield: 1 serving

Ingredients
½ cup of rolled oats
⅓ cup of unsweetened almond milk (or other non dairy milk)
3 tablespoons of pumpkin puree
2 teaspoons of pure maple syrup
½ teaspoon of vanilla extract
¼ teaspoon of ground cinnamon
A pinch of salt
Toasted pumpkin seeds or pecans, for garnish

Directions
Mix oats, milk, pumpkin, maple syrup, vanilla, cinnamon and salt in a jar that can hold a pint; stir well. Put a lid on and keep in the fridge overnight.

When you want to eat it, sprinkle pumpkin seeds (or pecans) on top, if you like.

Tips
You can do Step 1 and keep in the fridge for up to 4 days.

Oats that are labeled "gluten-free" should be used by people who have celiac disease or gluten-sensitivity, as wheat and barley often cross-contaminate oats.

Slow-Cooker Pasta e Fagioli Soup

Nutrition Facts || Fat **18g**, Carb **42g**, Protein **34g**, Fiber **8g**, Calories **457**
Prep Time: 15 mins, **Additional Time**: 8 hrs
Total Time: 8 hrs 15 mins, **Servings**: 6
Yield: 12 cups

Ingredients

2 cups of chopped onions

1 cup of chopped carrots

1 cup of chopped celery

1 pound of cooked Meal-Prep Sheet-Pan Chicken Thighs, diced

4 cups of cooked whole-wheat rotini pasta

6 cups of reduced-sodium chicken broth

4 teaspoons of dried Italian seasoning

¼ teaspoon of salt

1 (15 ounce) can of no-salt-added white beans, rinsed

4 cups of baby spinach (half of a 5-ounce box)

4 tablespoons of chopped fresh basil, divided (Optional)

2 tablespoons of best-quality extra-virgin olive oil

½ cup of grated Parmigiano-Reggiano cheese

Directions

Put onions, carrots and celery in a big plastic bag that can be sealed. Put cooked chicken and cooked pasta that have cooled down in another bag. Seal both bags and freeze for up to 5 days. Let the bags thaw in the fridge overnight before continuing.

Put the vegetable mixture in a big slow cooker. Add broth, Italian seasoning and salt. Cover and cook on Low for 7 ¼ hours.

Add beans, spinach, 2 tablespoons basil, if using, and the chicken and pasta that have thawed. Cook for 45 minutes more. Put the soup in bowls. Pour a little oil in each bowl and add cheese and the remaining 2 tablespoons basil, if you want.

Winter Vegetable Mulligatawny Soup

Nutrition Facts || Fat **15g**, Carb **76g**, Protein **14g**, Fiber **14g**, Calories **487**
Active Time: 25 mins, **Total Time**: 50 mins, **Servings**: 4
Yield: 4 servings

Ingredients

3 tablespoons of extra-virgin olive oil, divided

1 medium onion, finely chopped

2 medium carrots, finely chopped

1 medium parsnip, peeled and finely chopped

4 cups of peeled diced acorn squash or butternut squash

1 medium green apple, peeled and finely chopped

1 tablespoon of curry powder

3 cloves of garlic, minced, divided

1 teaspoon of grated fresh ginger

4 cups of low-sodium vegetable broth

1 (14 ounce) can of no-salt-added diced tomatoes

½ cup of red lentils, picked over and rinsed

2 whole-wheat naan flatbreads, halved

¼ cup of chopped fresh cilantro, plus more for garnish

Directions

Heat the oven to 375°F and cover a baking sheet with foil.

In a large saucepan, heat 2 tablespoons oil over medium heat until it sizzles. Put onion, carrots and parsnip in and cook until the onions are clear, about 6 minutes. Put squash, apple, curry powder, 2 cloves garlic and ginger in and cook, stirring, until it smells good, 1 to 2 minutes. Put broth, tomatoes and lentils in and stir to mix. Bring to a boil. Lower the heat to keep a low simmer, cover and cook until the squash and lentils are soft, about 20 minutes.

While that is cooking, brush one side of each naan with the remaining 1 tablespoon oil. Sprinkle with the remaining 1 clove garlic and put on the prepared baking sheet. Bake until warm, 5 to 6 minutes. Take out of oven and sprinkle with cilantro.

Mash some of the soup with a potato masher to make it as thick as you want. (Or, put half the soup in a blender and puree. Be careful when blending hot liquids.) Put cilantro on the soup and have it with the naan.

Tips
You can keep in the fridge for up to 4 days.

Lemony Linguine with Spring Vegetables

Nutrition Facts || Fat **7g**, Carb **64g**, Protein **18g**, Fiber **15g**, Calories **372**
Prep Time: 30 mins, **Total Time**: 30 mins, **Servings**: 4
Yield: 4 servings

Ingredients

8 ounces of whole-wheat linguine or fettuccine

4 cloves of garlic, thinly sliced

½ teaspoon of salt

¼ teaspoon of ground pepper

3 ½ cups of water

1 9-ounce of packaged frozen artichoke hearts

6 cups of chopped mature spinach

2 cups of peas, fresh or frozen

½ cup of grated Parmesan cheese, divided

¼ cup of half-and-half

1 tablespoon of lemon zest

3-4 tablespoons of lemon juice

Directions

In a large pot, mix pasta, garlic, salt and pepper. Pour water in. Bring to a boil over high heat. Boil, stirring often, for 8 minutes.

Add artichokes, spinach and peas and cook until the pasta is soft and the water is almost gone, 2 to 4 minutes more.

Take off the heat and stir in ¼ cup cheese, half-and-half, lemon zest and lemon juice as you like. Let it sit, stirring sometimes, for 5 minutes. Have it with the rest of the cheese on top.

Winter Kale & Quinoa Salad with Avocado

Nutrition Facts || Fat **20g**, Carb **54g**, Protein **15g**, Fiber **14g**, Calories **439**
Prep Time: 15 mins, **Additional Time**: 20mins
Total Time: 35 mins, **Servings**: 2
Yield: 2 servings

Ingredients

1 small sweet potato, peeled and cut into ½-inch pieces (1 ½ cups)
2 ½ teaspoons of olive oil, divided
½ avocado
1 tablespoon of lime juice
1 clove of garlic, peeled
½ teaspoon of ground cumin
⅛ teaspoon of salt
⅛ teaspoon of ground pepper
1-2 tablespoons of water
1 cup of cooked quinoa
¾ cup of no-salt-added canned black beans, rinsed
1 ½ cups of chopped baby kale
2 tablespoons of pepitas
1 scallion, chopped

Directions

Heat the oven to 400 degrees F and put sweet potato and 1 tsp. oil on a big baking sheet with edges. Bake, stirring once halfway, until soft, about 25 minutes.

In the meantime, put the rest of the oil, avocado, lime juice, garlic, cumin, salt, pepper, and 1 Tbsp. water in a blender or food processor and blend until smooth. Add 1 Tbsp. water if needed to make it as thin as you want.

Mix the sweet potato, quinoa, black beans, and kale in a medium bowl. Pour the avocado dressing over it and toss gently to coat. Sprinkle with pepitas and scallion.

Tips
Pepitas (pumpkin seeds without shells) can be found in the section with bulk foods in natural-foods stores and Mexican groceries.

Make sweet potato (Steps 1-2) and dressing (Step 3). You can keep them separate in the fridge for up to 2 days.

Addressing Common Challenges

Dealing with Cravings and Setbacks

Cravings can be hard to deal with when you want to have a heart-healthy lifestyle, but knowing what causes them and using effective ways can help you overcome these challenges.

Finding Out What Makes You Crave: Cravings often have specific reasons, such as emotions, situations, or foods. Finding out what makes you crave is the first step in dealing with cravings. Write down when cravings happen and any feelings or events that go along with them.

Healthy Choices: When cravings come, having DASH-friendly choices ready can make a big difference. For sweet cravings, try fresh fruit or a small amount of Greek yogurt with berries. For savory cravings, you can have air-popped popcorn or a handful of nuts.

Enjoying in Moderation: Instead of completely ignoring cravings, let yourself have small treats in a mindful way. Enjoying a small piece of dark chocolate or having a single serving of your favorite food can help you satisfy cravings without stopping your progress.

Drink Water: Sometimes thirst can be mistaken for hunger or cravings. Make sure you drink enough water by drinking water throughout the day, as this can help reduce unnecessary snack cravings.

Learn from Mistakes: Mistakes are part of any journey, and the key is to learn from them rather than seeing them as failures. Think about what caused the mistake, change your strategies if needed, and use it as a chance to grow.

Overcoming Obstacles to Adherence

The DASH Diet can be hard to stick to, but knowing and dealing with these challenges can make you stronger and achieve your goals.

Time Limits: A common challenge is the idea that following a healthy diet takes too much time. Overcome this by planning and preparing meals ahead of time. Cook in large batches on weekends or use kitchen tools that save time.

Social Expectations: Social events, especially those about food, can be hard. Tell your friends and family about your dietary choices, and don't be scared to stand up for them. Focus on the social part of events rather than just the food.

Limited Food Choices: Depending on where you are or what you have, you may not have many DASH-friendly foods. Look for local markets, try online grocery options, and get creative with different foods to overcome this challenge.

Emotional Eating: Emotional eating is a common challenge. Instead of eating food for comfort, find other ways to deal with emotions such as deep breathing, exercise, or doing a hobby.

Lack of Support: Having a support network is important. Be around people who understand and support your DASH goals. Think about joining online groups or forums to connect with people who share your interests.

Staying Motivated for Long-Term Success

Keeping motivation high for a long time is an important part of reaching lasting success on the DASH journey. Using effective ways can keep the fire of motivation alive.

Set Possible Goals: Make goals that you can achieve in the short term and the long term. Celebrate small wins along the way, and check and change goals as needed.

Think of Success: Imagine the benefits of reaching your DASH goals. Whether it's better health, more energy, or improved well-being, keeping these images in mind can boost motivation during hard times.

Make a Supportive Environment: Be around an environment that helps your DASH lifestyle. Have DASH-friendly foods in your kitchen, get rid of temptations, and create an atmosphere that matches your health goals.

Try Different Things: Keep interest in your food choices by trying different things in your meals. Find new recipes, eat different fruits and vegetables, and try different cooking methods to make things fun.

Check Regularly: Sometimes check your progress, think about what you have done, and recognize what you need to do better. This regular checking can help you stay involved and motivated on the DASH journey.

To deal with common challenges on the DASH Diet, you need a mixed approach, using self-awareness, strategic planning, and a strong mindset. By knowing and overcoming cravings, overcoming obstacles to following the diet, and keeping long-term motivation, people can not only adopt the DASH lifestyle but also achieve lasting success in their quest for heart-healthy living.

Answering Common Questions about the DASH Diet

Embarking on the DASH Diet often comes with a plethora of questions. Addressing these common queries provides clarity and empowers individuals to make informed choices.

1. What is the DASH Diet?
The DASH Diet is a dietary plan specifically designed to prevent and manage hypertension. It emphasizes whole, nutrient-dense foods such as fruits, vegetables, lean proteins, whole grains, and low-fat dairy while reducing sodium intake.

2. Is the DASH Diet Suitable for Weight Loss?
Yes, the DASH Diet is conducive to weight loss. Its emphasis on whole foods, portion control, and balanced nutrition can support weight management goals while promoting overall well-being.

3. Can I Follow the DASH Diet if I'm Vegetarian or Vegan?
Absolutely. The DASH Diet is flexible and can be adapted to various dietary preferences, including vegetarian and vegan lifestyles. Plant-based protein sources, such as legumes and tofu, can be incorporated to meet nutritional needs.

4. How Does the DASH Diet Affect Cholesterol Levels?
The DASH Diet's focus on heart-healthy fats, whole grains, and lean proteins contributes to improved cholesterol levels. By reducing saturated fat and cholesterol intake, individuals may experience positive changes in their lipid profiles.

5. Is Alcohol Allowed on the DASH Diet?

While moderate alcohol consumption is not explicitly restricted, it's advisable to limit alcohol intake. If consumed, it should be done in moderation, keeping in mind the additional calories and potential impact on blood pressure.

6. Is the DASH Diet Suitable for People with Diabetes?

Yes, the DASH Diet can be adapted for individuals with diabetes. Its emphasis on whole, nutrient-dense foods aligns well with diabetes management principles. However, it's advisable to consult with a healthcare professional for personalized guidance.

7. Can I Eat Out and Still Follow the DASH Diet?

Absolutely. When dining out, focus on choosing grilled or baked lean proteins, opting for vegetable sides, and being mindful of portion sizes. Ask for dressings and sauces on the side to control sodium intake.

8. How Fast Will I See Results on the DASH Diet?

The timeline for seeing results varies among individuals. Some may experience improvements in blood pressure within a few weeks, while others may take longer. Consistency in following the DASH principles is key to long-term success.

9. Is the DASH Diet Suitable for Children?

Yes, the DASH Diet can be adapted for children by ensuring age-appropriate portions and incorporating a variety of foods rich in nutrients. However, it's crucial to consult with a pediatrician or registered dietitian to tailor the diet to a child's specific needs.

10. Are Snacks Allowed on the DASH Diet?

Yes, snacks are allowed on the DASH Diet. Opt for nutrient-dense choices like fresh fruits, vegetables with hummus, Greek yogurt, or a handful of nuts. Be mindful of portion sizes to maintain the overall balance of your daily intake.

11. Is the DASH Diet Suitable for Pregnant Women?

The DASH Diet can be adapted for pregnant women with some modifications to ensure adequate nutrient intake. Consult with a healthcare provider or a registered dietitian to tailor the diet to meet specific prenatal needs.

12. Can I Use DASH for Weight Maintenance Once I Reach My Goal?

Yes, the DASH Diet can be a sustainable choice for weight maintenance. Transitioning to a modified DASH plan that aligns with your energy needs can help you sustain the benefits achieved during weight loss.

13. How Does DASH Address Specific Nutritional Needs for Different Age Groups?

The DASH Diet can be adapted for various age groups by adjusting portion sizes and nutrient requirements. Children, adolescents, adults, and older adults can all benefit from the foundational principles of the DASH Diet.

14. Is DASH Suitable for Athletes or Those with High Physical Activity Levels?

Absolutely. Athletes and individuals with high physical activity levels can adapt the DASH Diet to meet their energy needs. Emphasizing nutrient-dense foods and adjusting portion sizes based on activity levels is key.

15. Are Artificial Sweeteners Allowed on the DASH Diet?

While the DASH Diet doesn't explicitly restrict artificial sweeteners, it encourages moderation. It's advisable to choose natural sweeteners like honey or maple syrup in limited amounts and be mindful of their impact on overall nutrition.

16. Can I Use DASH if I Have Food Allergies or Sensitivities?

Yes, the DASH Diet is adaptable to various dietary needs, including allergies or sensitivities. Modify recipes and food choices based on your specific requirements, and consult with a healthcare professional or dietitian for personalized guidance.

17. Is the DASH Diet Suitable for Individuals with Kidney Issues?

The DASH Diet can often be modified for individuals with kidney issues, but it's essential to consult with a healthcare provider or a renal dietitian for personalized recommendations. Adjustments in protein and potassium intake may be necessary.

18. How Can I Make DASH Kid-Friendly for Picky Eaters?

Introduce DASH-friendly foods gradually, involve children in meal planning and preparation, and get creative with presentations. Incorporate flavors and textures that appeal to their tastes while maintaining the nutritional integrity of the DASH Diet.

19. Can I Follow DASH as a Vegan or Vegetarian Athlete?

Absolutely. Vegan and vegetarian athletes can meet their nutrient needs by choosing plant-based protein sources, incorporating a variety of colorful fruits and vegetables, and ensuring adequate intake of essential nutrients. Consult with a dietitian for personalized advice.

20. What Snacks Can I Have on the DASH Diet?

DASH-friendly snacks include fresh fruit, raw vegetables with hummus, Greek yogurt, a small handful of nuts, or whole-grain crackers with cheese. The key is to choose nutrient-dense options in appropriate portions.

Solutions to Common Challenges and Misconceptions

Navigating challenges and dispelling misconceptions is integral to a successful DASH experience. Here are solutions to common hurdles encountered on the DASH journey.

1. Challenge: Feeling Deprived

Solution: Embrace the abundance of delicious, nutrient-packed foods the DASH Diet offers. Experiment with new recipes, flavors, and cooking techniques to keep meals exciting.

2. Challenge: High Sodium Levels in Processed Foods

Solution: Be vigilant about reading food labels and choose low-sodium or sodium-free alternatives. Cooking at home with fresh ingredients allows for better control over salt intake.

3. Challenge: Difficulty Adhering to Daily Servings

Solution: Plan meals in advance, create a weekly menu, and batch-cook when possible. This helps ensure that you have DASH-friendly options readily available.

4. Challenge: Limited Time for Meal Preparation

Solution: Embrace quick and easy DASH-friendly recipes. Prepping ingredients in advance, utilizing time-saving kitchen tools, and incorporating leftovers into future meals can streamline the cooking process.

5. Challenge: Social Pressure to Conform to Unhealthy Eating Habits

Solution: Communicate your dietary preferences to friends and family, and explain the health benefits of the DASH Diet. Encourage them to join you on the journey or be supportive of your choices.

6. Challenge: Traveling While Following the DASH Diet

Solution: Plan ahead by researching local restaurants with DASH-friendly options, pack nutritious snacks, and choose wisely when dining out. Consider bringing portable items like nuts, seeds, and dried fruits.

7. Challenge: Managing DASH on a Budget

Solution: Optimize your grocery budget by purchasing affordable staple foods in bulk, choosing seasonal produce, and exploring cost-effective protein sources like legumes and eggs.

8. Challenge: Balancing DASH with Specific Cultural or Dietary Preferences

Solution: Modify traditional recipes to align with DASH principles. Choose lean proteins, whole grains, and plenty of vegetables. Experiment with herbs and spices to enhance flavors without compromising nutritional integrity.

9. Challenge: Maintaining DASH During Special Occasions or Holidays**

Solution: Plan ahead for events by contributing DASH-friendly dishes, practicing portion control, and focusing on social aspects rather than solely on the food. Make informed choices without feeling deprived.

10. Challenge: Balancing DASH with a Busy Lifestyle

Solution: Dedicate time for weekly meal planning and prep to ensure DASH-friendly meals are readily available. Explore quick and simple DASH recipes that fit into a busy schedule. Keep DASH-friendly snacks on hand for busy days.

11. Misconception: DASH is Only for Individuals with Hypertension

Solution: While the DASH Diet is designed to manage and prevent hypertension, its principles contribute to overall heart health and can be adopted by anyone interested in a balanced, nutritious diet.

12. Misconception: DASH is Restrictive and Bland

Solution: Explore the vast array of DASH-friendly recipes that showcase diverse flavors and culinary styles. The diet is not about restriction but about enjoying a variety of nutrient-rich foods.

13. Misconception: DASH Requires Elimination of All Fats

Solution: DASH encourages healthy fats, such as those found in olive oil, avocados, and nuts. These fats are an essential part of a balanced diet and contribute to overall cardiovascular health.

14. Misconception: DASH is a Short-Term Solution

Solution: The DASH Diet is not a quick-fix solution. It is a sustainable, long-term approach to promoting heart health and overall well-being. Embrace it as a lifestyle rather than a temporary diet.

15. Misconception: All Carbohydrates are Restricted on the DASH Diet

Solution: The DASH Diet encourages whole grains and complex carbohydrates. Include sources like brown rice, quinoa, and whole wheat bread in moderation for a balanced intake of macronutrients.

16. Misconception: DASH Requires Significant Financial Investment

Solution: The DASH Diet can be affordable. Focus on seasonal produce, buy in bulk when possible, and choose cost-effective protein sources. Planning meals in advance also helps minimize waste.

17. Misconception: DASH is Only About Sodium Reduction

Solution: While sodium reduction is a key focus, the DASH Diet encompasses a broader approach, emphasizing a balanced intake of nutrients. Focus on the variety of whole, nutrient-dense foods that contribute to heart health.

18. Misconception: DASH is Too Complex to Follow

Solution: Start by incorporating small changes. Gradually introduce DASH-friendly foods and explore simple recipes. As you become more familiar with the principles, you can expand your repertoire.

19. Misconception: DASH is One-Size-Fits-All

Solution: The DASH Diet is adaptable. Tailor it to your individual needs, preferences, and health goals. Consulting with a healthcare professional or registered dietitian can provide personalized guidance.

20. Misconception: DASH Requires Complete Elimination of Processed Foods

Solution: While minimizing processed foods is encouraged, complete elimination is not necessary. Be discerning in your choices, and opt for minimally processed options when available.

21. Misconception: DASH is Only for Older Adults

Solution: The DASH Diet is suitable for individuals of all ages. Its principles promote heart health and overall well-being, making it a valuable dietary approach for anyone interested in preventive health measures.

22. Misconception: DASH Doesn't Allow for Flavorful Meals

Solution: The DASH Diet embraces' a variety of herbs, spices, and other flavor-enhancing ingredients. Explore different culinary techniques and ingredients to create delicious, flavorful meals while adhering to DASH principles.

23. Misconception: DASH Requires Drastic Dietary Changes

Solution: Gradual changes are effective. Start by incorporating one or two DASH principles at a time. As these become habits, progressively introduce additional aspects of the diet for a sustainable transition.

24. Misconception: DASH is Only About Restriction

Solution: Focus on the abundance of nutrient-dense foods that the DASH Diet encourages. Emphasize the positive aspects of the diet, such as increased energy, improved well-being, and a reduced risk of heart disease.

25. Misconception: DASH is Only for People with Hypertension

Solution: The DASH Diet extends beyond hypertension, promoting heart health, weight management, and overall well-being. Its nutrient-rich approach supports individuals of all ages, offering a flexible and sustainable dietary lifestyle. Dispelling this misconception involves raising awareness about the broader benefits of DASH and integrating its principles into public health initiatives for a comprehensive approach to optimal health.

By addressing an array of questions and challenges associated with the DASH Diet, individuals can tailor this heart-healthy approach to their specific needs, preferences, and lifestyles. Staying informed, seeking support, and adopting a flexible mindset contribute to the successful integration of the DASH lifestyle.

Beyond the Basics

Integrating DASH into a Holistic Lifestyle

Adopting DASH into your lifestyle means embracing a holistic view of health. It is not only about following dietary guidelines, but also about being mindful of how you eat, staying physically active, managing stress, and getting enough quality sleep. These factors complement each other to form a comprehensive health strategy, emphasizing the interdependence of lifestyle habits.

Action Steps:
1. Eat mindfully by enjoying each bite and appreciating the nourishment it provides.
2. Choose physical activities that you like, which will improve your heart health and overall fitness.
3. Try stress-relieving activities such as meditation, yoga, or hobbies that make you happy and relaxed.

4. Make sure you get enough and restful sleep, knowing that it has a significant impact on your heart health.

Combining DASH with Other Healthy Habits

DASH works better when combined with other healthy habits. These habits include drinking enough water, avoiding tobacco and limiting alcohol, which all support the DASH lifestyle. By following a comprehensive approach, you can strengthen your dedication to heart health.

Action Steps:
1. Drink enough water throughout the day to stay hydrated.
2. Stop smoking and stay away from secondhand smoke, which can harm your heart.
3. Limit alcohol intake, following DASH and general health guidelines.
4. Check your blood pressure and other health measures regularly to see your progress and make changes if needed.

Long-Term Strategies for Heart Health

Keeping your heart healthy requires long-term strategies that are more than just short-term dietary changes. DASH is a solid foundation, but you need to be persistent and flexible to integrate it into your lifestyle. This section discusses the principles of a heart-healthy life, emphasizing the permanent nature of these practices.

Action Steps:
1. Have a positive outlook on health, treating it as an ongoing journey rather than a destination.
2. Adapt to the evolving nature of nutrition by staying updated on research and making adjustments to your dietary choices.

3. Build a supportive environment by joining a community that shares similar health goals.

4. Seek advice from healthcare professionals frequently to ensure customized guidance that suits your evolving health needs.

In essence, going beyond the basics of the DASH Diet involves weaving its principles into the fabric of your daily life. It's about creating a sustainable and enriching lifestyle that prioritizes heart health while recognizing the intricate interplay of various well-being factors. By embracing a holistic approach, you can elevate your overall quality of life and enjoy the enduring benefits of a heart-healthy lifestyle.

Tips from those who successfully incorporated DASH into their lives

Learning from the wisdom of those who have successfully made DASH part of their lifestyles offers valuable insights for others on a similar path. These tips include practical advice on meal planning, handling social situations, and staying motivated. The collective wisdom of successful DASH practitioners provides a guide for newcomers seeking to make lasting changes.

Expert Tips:

1. "Begin slowly by adding one DASH principle at a time. Small, consistent changes lead to lasting results."

2. "Try new recipes to keep meals interesting. DASH isn't about restriction but about enjoying a variety of nutrient-rich foods."

3. "Find a support system. Whether it's friends, family, or an online community, having others on the same journey can be incredibly motivating."

4. "Be consistent with the DASH principles. It's the daily, small choices that add up to create lasting change. Don't let occasional slips discourage you; just get back on track."

5. "Have fun with it! Experiment with herbs, spices, and different cooking methods. DASH isn't about boring meals; it's about discovering the rich flavors of wholesome ingredients."

6. "Don't forget to hydrate! Add fruits or herbs to water for a refreshing twist. Staying well-hydrated supports the DASH Diet and contributes to overall health."

7. "Eat mindfully. Slow down, savor each bite, and pay attention to your body's hunger and fullness cues. It transforms meals into a holistic experience."
8. "Prepare ahead of time. Have DASH-friendly snacks and meals ready to go. It reduces the temptation of reaching for less healthy options when you're hungry and pressed for time."

9. "Remember, DASH is more than just what's on your plate. Embrace stress-reducing activities, prioritize quality sleep, and celebrate the holistic lifestyle that DASH promotes."

10. "Listen to your body. It communicates with you. If certain foods make you feel energized and vibrant, take note. It's about creating a personalized, sustainable approach that suits your unique needs."

11. "Share your DASH journey. Whether it's with friends, family, or online communities, connecting with others on a similar path provides support, inspiration, and valuable insights.

12. "Social situations can be challenging, but they don't have to derail your progress. Learn to navigate restaurant menus, choose wisely at gatherings, and show others that heart-healthy choices can be delicious and satisfying."

13. "Celebrate more than just the numbers on the scale. Recognize the non-scale victories – increased energy, better sleep, and an overall sense of well-being. These are the true markers of success."

Success Stories; Real-life accounts of individuals benefiting from the DASH Diet

The best way to appreciate the power of the DASH Diet is through the real-life experiences of individuals who have embraced its principles. Personal stories illustrate the challenges faced, the motivations that drove a commitment to DASH, and the remarkable outcomes achieved. From lowering blood pressure to shedding weight and gaining more energy, these stories demonstrate the different ways DASH has enhanced lives.

Mary's Story: A Victory Over High Blood Pressure

Mary is a 52-year-old woman who experienced a significant change in her life when she learned about the amazing power of the DASH Diet. She had high blood pressure and decided to take control of her health. She realized that she needed to make lasting changes and followed the DASH principles.

In the first few months, Mary faced the challenge of adapting to a new way of eating. However, with perseverance and a gradual approach, she added more fruits, vegetables, and whole grains to her meals. Over time, Mary saw a remarkable change in her blood pressure readings. The numbers started to normalize, and her energy levels increased.

Mary's success story is more than just lowering her blood pressure. She developed a new appreciation for tasty and nutritious foods. DASH became not just a dietary plan but a lifestyle that Mary adopted with enthusiasm. Now, she shares her story to inspire others, emphasizing that it's never too late to take charge of one's health.

John's Transformation: A Weight Loss Success

John, at 35, found himself at a point where he wanted to make a lasting change in his life. He was overweight and aware of his family history of high blood pressure, so he chose the DASH Diet. John's journey was not only about losing weight but adopting a sustainable approach to health.

His before-and-after story shows a clear picture of transformation. The 'before' image showed a man burdened by unhealthy habits, while the 'after' radiated health and well-being. John credits his weight loss success to a consistent adherence to DASH principles, focusing on portion control and nutrient-rich foods.

John's journey went beyond the physical realm. He discovered a new joy in preparing and enjoying meals. DASH not only helped him achieve a healthier weight but also cultivated a positive relationship with food. John's story resonates with those seeking a holistic approach to well-being, proving that DASH is not just a diet but a catalyst for a healthier, happier life.

Susan's Lifestyle Revolution with DASH

Susan, at 45, approached the DASH Diet with a unique perspective – not as a temporary fix but as a lifestyle revolution. Her journey was marked by a desire for sustained well-being and a departure from restrictive diets. Susan's story unfolds as a testament to the enduring nature of DASH principles.

Before DASH, Susan faced the typical challenges of modern life – stress, occasional unhealthy eating, and fluctuating energy levels. DASH became her anchor, providing a framework for balanced nutrition and a foundation for overall health. The 'before' image depicted a woman navigating the complexities of a busy life, while the 'after' showcased a picture of resilience, energy, and vitality.

Susan's tips for success include finding joy in the journey, experimenting with diverse recipes, and creating a supportive network. Her story resonates with those seeking a sustainable and enjoyable approach to health, emphasizing that DASH is not just about managing blood pressure but fostering a lifestyle that promotes long-term well-being.

In the realm of the DASH Diet, success stories serve as beacons of inspiration. They illustrate the transformative potential of embracing heart-healthy practices and provide a roadmap for others seeking similar positive changes. Through real-life accounts, before-and-after narratives, and practical tips, this section celebrates the achievements of individuals who have not only adopted the DASH Diet but have also redefined their lives in the process.

Recap of Key DASH Principles

As we conclude this exploration into the Dietary Approaches to Stop Hypertension (DASH), it's time to revisit the key principles that form the bedrock of this heart-healthy lifestyle. This section encapsulates the essence of DASH, recapping its foundational principles and offering words of encouragement for a future steeped in heart health.

The journey through the DASH Diet has been a holistic experience, encompassing more than just dietary changes. Let's revisit the fundamental principles that have guided us:

1. Fruits and Vegetables: The vibrant colors of fruits and vegetables have been our allies, providing essential vitamins, minerals, and antioxidants.

2. Lean Proteins: From poultry to legumes, incorporating lean protein sources has been central to maintaining muscle health and satiety.

3. Whole Grains: Whole grains have been the cornerstone of energy, supplying fiber and nutrients for sustained vitality.

4. Low-Fat Dairy: A commitment to low-fat dairy has fortified our bones and contributed to overall nutritional balance.

5. Moderation in Sodium: Conscious choices to limit sodium intake have played a crucial role in managing blood pressure and supporting cardiovascular health.

6. Balanced Portion Control: Understanding portion sizes has empowered us to enjoy a variety of foods while maintaining balance and preventing overconsumption.

Encouragement for a Heart-Healthy Future

As you stand at the intersection of your DASH journey, envision a future where heart health is not just a goal but a way of life. Your commitment to these principles is an investment in a thriving tomorrow. Let these words of encouragement guide your path:

Embrace Progress, Not Perfection:
- The DASH journey is a continual process of growth. Celebrate your progress, no matter how small, and remember that each positive choice contributes to your overall well-being.

Cherish the Joy of Nourishing Your Body:
- Approach meals with gratitude and joy. Nourishing your body is an act of self-love. Let the flavors of wholesome foods bring delight to your palate and fulfillment to your heart.

Forge a Supportive Community:
- Share your DASH journey with others. Whether it's family, friends, or an online community, building a support system enhances your resilience and keeps you inspired.

Embody a Heart-Healthy Lifestyle:
- Beyond the plate, let the principles of DASH permeate every facet of your life. Engage in regular physical activity, manage stress, prioritize quality sleep, and revel in the holistic benefits of a heart-healthy lifestyle.

Celebrate Your Commitment:
- Your commitment to DASH is a celebration of self-care and longevity. As you navigate life's journey, let your heart-healthy choices be a beacon, guiding you toward a future filled with vitality and well-being.

In conclusion, the DASH Diet is not merely a set of guidelines but a blueprint for a heart-healthy lifestyle. May your journey be filled with discovery, resilience, and the unwavering belief that you hold the power to shape a future where your heart beats with vibrancy and strength. Here's to a heart-healthy tomorrow and the endless possibilities it brings, Cheers!

Your Feedback Matters

Dear Readers,

I hope this message finds you well. I am reaching out to express my sincere gratitude for choosing to read "DASH Delights". Your support means the world to me, and I genuinely hope the book has been an enjoyable and insightful experience for you.

As an author, reader reviews are incredibly important, not just for me but for fellow readers who might be considering this book. Your honest feedback can make a significant difference in helping others discover the value within these pages.

If you could spare a few moments to share your thoughts on "DASH Delights" whether on Amazon, Goodreads or elsewhere, it would be immensely appreciated. Feel free to share your insights on what resonated with you, any favorite parts, or how the book may have impacted you.

Your reviews contribute not only to the visibility of the book but also help me understand the aspects that readers find most valuable. Your honest perspective is invaluable, and I am genuinely looking forward to hearing your thoughts.

Thank you once again for being a part of this journey. Your support and feedback mean everything.

Warm regards,
Leopold Knight

Culinary Adventures with Leopold Knight

Dear Readers,

Allow me to extend my deepest gratitude for joining me on the culinary journey through "DASH Delights." It's been a pleasure sharing my passion for health-conscious and delectable cuisine with you.

If "DASH Delights" left your taste buds craving more, I'm thrilled to invite you to explore additional culinary adventures scheduled to be released in "Leopold's Healthy Diet" series of which "DASH Delights" is the second book.

The first book titled "Easy Dog Food Recipes Cookbook for Beginners" which is for dog enthusiasts is a comprehensive guide to homemade dog food recipes and canine nutrition for nourishing your furry friend.

Discover My Author Central Page:
Curious about the inspiration behind the recipes and the informational guide? Visit my Author Central Page to delve deeper into the culinary universe. Here, you'll find behind-the-scenes glimpses, upcoming releases, and a space where readers and food enthusiasts connect. Follow the link or scan the QR code to connect to my Author Central Page.

www.amazon.com/author/leopoldknight

Leopold Knight's Culinary Philosophy:

My journey as a chef is not just about recipes; it's a celebration of the beautiful connection between flavorful dishes and a healthier lifestyle. From the kitchen to your table, I strive to create meals that nourish both the body and the spirit. Your ongoing support and engagement mean the world to me. Thank you for being a part of this flavorful adventure. I look forward to continuing to share the joy of cooking and healthy living with you.

Sincerely,
Leopold Knight